I took but a millisecond to spring from the bed to the closet and retrieve my pistol from its holster.

She sat on the bed watching, her eyes both loathing me and cheering me on: "Do it! Do it and get it over with!"

I placed the .32 at that point just behind my right ear that would guarantee an instant death as the small projectile tore its way through bone, brain, and other assorted tissue. I felt the oncoming surge of momentum that would end in an explosion that I would never hear.

For a split second in time I was an un-person. No pain, hurt, sorrow, or regret. No joy or laughter, no feeling of existence. I saw dear friends flash by in microseconds. I saw myself making a promise that I was about to break in the most violent way.

I did not feel the weight of the gun at my head. Only the slow, consistent pressure on the trigger. *Remember, never jerk the trigger of your weapon; squeeze it with steady pressure. When the weapon fires, it should be a surprise to you.* The pressure was on the trigger. I awaited my surprise.

To Pat

TEARS OF BLOOD

The Betrayal of America's Veterans

Welcome Home
We got a lot to do to make
things right again
Best Wishes

CHUCK LAWRENCE

Chuck

SOARING EAGLE

PUBLISHING

Auburn, Washington

SOARING EAGLE PUBLISHING COMPANY
P.O. Box 2536
Auburn, Washington 98071-2536
Copyright © 1998 by Chuck Lawrence

TEARS OF BLOOD
The Betrayal of America's Veterans

ISBN 0-9659743-0-8 (paperback)
ISBN 0-9659743-9-1 (hardcover)
Library of Congress Catalog Card Number: 97-80994

First edition

All rights reserved. Except for review and citations not exceeding 50 words, no portion of this book may be reproduced by any means without permission of the author or publisher

For permission to quote, cite, or reprint, or to arrange a teaching, speaking, or events engagement with the author, write the publisher or E-mail:

Y34@aol.com

This book is a work of biographical nonfiction. All persons, places, and events in this book are entirely true, but all names have been changed to protect privacy. However, except for the names which appear on the transcript of the ABC-TV News presentation, 20/20, and the names of United States Presidents and their Cabinet members, all characters in this story have been given fictitious names to protect individuals' identity and privacy.

Cover design by Andrea Fitcha

Layout and book design by DIMI PRESS

Dedicated to Ron Beck

I never knew you as a person, Ron. You were a short blurb on a television newsmagazine show. You were a man, a soldier, a veteran who was let down by the country you so proudly served.

But for a moment in time, I would have met your fate ... but I remembered: I remembered a promise I made to you when I saw your story. I remembered you and you did not allow me to do what I would have done had I not felt your presence. I rode the same razor's edge that you were on, but because of you I got off and took a different direction.

I hope your personal sacrifice will live through what I am trying to accomplish with this book. I hope I will help others as your story helped me.

Rest in peace, my Brother

ACKNOWLEDGEMENTS

While the writing of this book proved to be a major catharsis for me personally, there are many without whom I would never have completed this work.

Richie Gough, Henry Rossic, and the other members of VVA Chapter 12 who gave me the original idea and were there when I needed them most.

Col. Beau Bergereon (Ret), director of the Washington State Department of Veterans Affairs, with whom I have had the privilege of working on many veterans issues. Beau is a real veteran in the purest sense. After reading the original manuscript, Beau gave me the courage to pursue this project.

Bill Landry (USCG Ret), who helped turn a real mess of a manuscript into something that makes a little sense.

Zack and Jenine Heitz, two very special friends who stood with me, not only through the writing of the book but while I dealt with personal crises, struggles, and fears. You believed in me and in this book from the very outset. Without your wisdom and confidence this surely would never have come to pass.

Mike Murphy, who would not allow me to let this project die. Mike, you have been that bit of shining light that brings brightness to a dark world ... but then, you and I have a special bond that can not be erased by time, distance, or circumstance.

My sister, Eva, who, during the final production of this work, was senselessly murdered. Sis, I know we talked about how the completion of this work would have made things a lot better for you and your son. You led a hard life, but you managed with dignity and an inner strength that is rare in this world today. God bless you.

Special thanks to Devereux Chatillon and ABC-TV for permission to reprint the copyrighted transcript of "Whose Side Are They On?" from ABC News 20/20, October 2, 1987.

Many others have been there and supported me in this project: friends, associates, fellow veterans, many knowing full well how emotional and sometimes embarrassing it is to open one's life as I have. To all of you—you know who you are—thank you.

INTRODUCTION

Like so many of us who proudly served our country in Vietnam, Chuck Lawrence was greeted by bureaucratic structures like the U.S. Department of Veterans Affairs (formerly the Veterans Administration) which were unresponsive, crass, and extremely difficult to deal with. The DVA did not fulfill its role of veterans' advocate as mandated by federal law.

Chuck has written a compelling account of his experience with the DVA. He masterfully identifies how the agency's lethargy adversely impacted his family and ultimately caused even more trauma than his distinguished combat service in Southeast Asia.

Tears of Blood describes in vivid detail the workings of the VA system, and tells Americans that their tax dollars dedicated to assist veterans are misused. While Chuck identifies the numerous problems in this sluggish and unresponsive system, he also presents solutions to correct them.

Tears of Blood conveys with unique passion the trials and tribulations of a terribly wronged Vietnam veteran and the daunting problems of "the system" — problems which not only need to be highlighted, but need to be fixed. The book is not written with malice but with the more noble intent of helping our country's 27 million veterans by showing them how the system has failed them. And it conveys a lucid message to our nation's future military personnel.

This book distinguishes itself from previous works by effectively addressing a subject which has not heretofore appeared in print. It goes beyond the war to focus on how the situations of post-discharge amplify problems like Post Traumatic Stress Disorder and other war-related traumas.

Tears of Blood is compelling reading. Equally important, Chuck's story provides an avenue for self-healing for all veterans who have experienced not only the hardships of combat, but the difficulties associated with accessing the VA system.

Get set for a fast-paced, hard-slamming, direct-hit story, told on a roller-coaster ride of human emotions.

Colonel A.J. "Beau" Bergeron (USA-Ret.)
Director, Washington State Department of Veterans Affairs
First Cavalry Platoon Leader, Vietnam 1966-67
Armored Cavalry Troop Commander, Vietnam 1969-70

Poor is the country that has no Heroes But Beggared is that people who having them, **FORGET!**

UNKNOWN

FOREWORD

When any nation calls upon its youth and its military to take action with force of arms, that nation has a responsibility to those men and women who answer the call. It matters not the reason for the sounding of the bugles and the beating of the drums. It matters not if the soldier or sailor or pilot is a volunteer or a draftee, whether the bearing of arms is a career or a one-time duty. It matters not the gender nor any other ascribed delineation. The fact is men and women serve and place themselves in harm's way for the good of our nation, as directed by the Commander in Chief and defined by our Congress. In doing so the Commander in Chief and the Congress assume responsibility to those who serve.

It is incumbent upon a nation to ensure that such obligation is indeed honored. Whether in time of war or peace, the nation owes a debt to those who protect it. Promises to care for those injured or debilitated by illness or condition in the line of duty must be absolute and unconditional. It is the least a nation can do for its protectors and defenders.

If the nation and its leaders do not fulfill their obligation to care for its fallen, who would be willing to serve? Our citizens must be able to enter the military with the absolute knowledge that if they are disabled while in the line of duty, they will be cared for. They must know that if their injuries are permanent and affect their lives, they will continue to be cared for and justly compensated.

For decades, our national leaders, our legislators and our representatives have made such promises. The United States Department of Veterans Affairs was formed to meet the needs of our injured and disabled. Unfortunately, budget cuts, attitudes, and bureaucratic apathy have wreaked havoc with the system and annihilated the faith of those who are supposed to be served. Budgets and deficits are used to disguise incompetence and disdain for the people. Social programs accelerate at a carcinogous rate while those who defend this nation (and the rest of the world) are left to fend for themselves.

Former enemies whom our military once stood against get *carte blanche* in the form of refugee status. A third of America's homeless are veterans who once proudly served this nation but are reduced to scraping out a survival in our inner cities. Betrayal and poverty create criminals out of heroes. More Vietnam veterans have committed suicide than were killed in that war.

Troops' exposure to untested chemicals, to Agent Orange, Blue, and to nuclear materials continues to destroy the veteran's mind, health, body ... family, work; his spirit. Rather than bureaucrats' accepting that something is very wrong, they cloak themselves in excuses and denial. Not all these problems have simple and concrete answers — but many do.
It is called *justice*. It can be achieved when the nation honors its word to those that serve.

This book is my story. A story of years of denials and crass attitudes and apathy by the very agency legislated to serve me. It kept me under its heel. It prevented me from being the productive citizen I tried to be. It cost me a family I dearly loved. And yes, it added my name for a time to the list of homeless.

Veterans service organizations are wrapped in the Washington, D.C. "Beltway mentality," forgetting who and what they are there to represent, ignoring what they are there to accomplish. Service organizations are supposed to protect veterans' rights. Instead, they set up their own hierarchies, write their own agendas, and rule themselves according to personal egos, individuals' hunger for power, and internal politics. The bureaucrat becomes *Numero Uno*.

We as a nation can ill afford this apathy and incompetence, for one day we shall be repaid for it. What happens when no one chooses to serve because they who serve are the despised and our nation's promises are meaningless?

Yes, this book chronicles one man's personal story; but it also is the story of thousands of others who have died, or simply gave up the struggle and disappeared into the alleys and doorways or the screaming silence of derangement. It is also the story of the few who continue to struggle for the fulfillment of the promises made to them when they went off to fight an enemy they didn't know in a country they never heard of for a cause that was not clear — but who did so believing that God would bless America.

It is time to make this nation understand that the Department of Veterans Affairs is there to honor — it *must* honor — its moral and legal obligations to those who serve. The VA is not a welfare office, though many who never wore a uniform believe it is.

Let this book be a call to all veterans to come together, united. Let this be our cause: To demand the fulfillment of the promises made to us, to finally be granted the rights which are guaranteed by the faith of a nation. Let us not allow that nation's word to be meaningless.

Chuck Lawrence
1998

PART ONE

1

In 1981 I was discharged from the United States Army—for the second time. I was reluctant, afraid.

I did not want to leave the military. For twelve and a half years the Army had been my career. Hell, it was my whole life; that and my wife Tina—my friend, my pillar and rock.

I feared being out of the Army. Still, almost ten years later, Vietnam nagged and haunted me. We returning Nam vets were not the most desirable or accepted part of society and I couldn't adjust to the scorn. What would it be like now in the eighties, I worried.

My first discharge was in 1972, after two tours in Vietnam. When I returned from there, I discovered that the American people neither wanted nor liked nor supported that war, and those of us who fought it were the despised ones.

"Impressive qualifications, Mr. Smith / Brown / Hatachi / O'McMurphy / Goschanowicz. You'll be a tremendous asset to our . . . What's this? Vietnam? Gee, I'm sorry; we are not hiring at this time."

Then there was Gary, a draftee kid who earned a Bronze Star and a Purple Heart. The day after Gary arrived home from Nam, he walked the streets of one of those bergs whose major economy was its protesting, anti-government, flag-burning, draft-dodging, liberal hippie university students. After forty minutes on the city streets Gary had to duck into the first department store to buy an entire new change of clothes because the uniform he wore was soaking wet with the spit from passing-by citizens he had defended, and stained with the soil of assorted items hurled at him from local trash cans.

Personally, I couldn't deal with the public's hostility. I got my honorable discharge after being severely injured in Nam, I tried the go-to-college bit, tried to get a job and simply go to work. I was not wanted. So I returned to the army and chose it as my career and future. It was a comfortable sanctuary; there I didn't have to keep trying to hide the fact that I had served in that miserable excuse of a war.

During my second enlistment I was an instructor in the Infantry Officer's Basic Course at Ft. Benning, Georgia. When, in December, 1979, I was leveled flat by an intestinal disturbance, I thought I must have chowed down on some bad food during field training. It turned out to be more than just a stomach ache; on New Years Eve my wife rushed me to the post hospital. I ended up spending a whole month there, wired up to all kinds of bottles and tubes.

After I left the hospital I figured that with enough self-discipline I could hide the fact that I was seriously ailing. Not well enough, though; within weeks the commandant removed me from my field command. I had never *not* been in the field, and not being there left me unsettled and disoriented. I am a field grunt, not a Garrison Troopie!

"I'm pretty sure you have Crohn's disease," my doctor said. "But that's only a preliminary diagnosis. We can't be certain until the disease has more time to assert itself."

"Crohn's disease?" I asked. "What is that?"

"A serious disorder of the intestinal system."

"How will it effect me?"

"It isn't a pretty disease, Chuck. Crohn's suffers go through periods when they can't assimilate food. Symptoms are cramps, pain, chronic diarrhea, rectal bleeding, lethargy, weight loss, and control problems."

I pressed on. "What's the cure? How long will I have it? Does it get worse?"

The doc hesitated. "Well ... we don't have a cure, so far. Medication, to relieve the pain. Sometimes you can control it with a bland liquid diet. The episodes come and go, but over time the disease progresses and worsens."

I sat there saying nothing, trying to let the information soak in.

Quickly the doctor added, "But that's only a preliminary diagnosis. We can't be certain until the disease has more to assert itself. Let's see you every other week for the time being, just to track things. But come in immediately any time you think you're having any kind of digestive problem."

But the Army lives to transfer soldiers. My doctor was sent to Texas and I was in Germany before he got to finish the diagnosis. That lack of a completed diagnosis was to bring me to the brink of ruin, to the very edge of death, over the next ten years.

In Germany, where I was transferred from the Infantry to my new position as a communications platoon sergeant, I could not get the specialized treatment I needed. In fact the military doctors there gave me no attention at all even though my condition steadily worsened. I had chronic diarrhea, I was in constant pain, and the doctors offered me no relief. I would work for two or three days then be in bed for the next three. That was unfair to the men in my platoon who counted on me for leadership and guidance.

"Leave the Army, Chuck," Tina said, clasping her hands protectively around the barely-beginning-to-show swell that silently announced she was carrying our first child.

"Yeah, sure. Me with my GED and my twelve and a half years' work experience as a combat soldier and field trainer, with medical problems, and a family to support."

"The VA will take care of your Crohn's Disease—"

"It hasn't been completely and officially diagnosed."

"But it *is* Crohn's. As soon as you're discharged the VA will get you a decent doctor and it'll be properly diagnosed. And I'll get a job while you go to school to learn a civilian skill. Then it'll be my turn to go to college. First you go to school while I work, then you work while I go to school."

The United States Army granted my request for an honorable discharge and, on January 15, 1981, I again became an ex-soldier.

My balance book carried two assets of great wealth: my confidence in myself, and one hell of a woman's total support. On the other side of the ledger, though, was fear. I feared the civilian community would scorn a Nam vet the same way it did in 1971, and I was sure none could understand the ghosts that still haunted me even though the war was ten years past. I knew I wouldn't be able to talk to anyone about it, because no one cared, much less understood.

Hours after my discharge we arrived at my parents' home on the outskirts of Seattle. From their garage I retrieved my '68 Mustang and Tina and I flanked out in two directions, each of us concentrating on separate tasks to establish ourselves in civilian life. My wife began the search for a doctor and a birthing place for our baby, and for a home to take it to. I began the search for a college and a yet undecided course of study, and commenced filling out forms for Veterans Administration registration and more forms for unemployment benefits.

The first place I honored by my presence was the Washington State Division of . . . is it Employment, or Unemployment? I wanted to begin receiving unemployment benefits as soon as possible, but I wanted even more to become employed. Anyway, it was supposed to be a one-stop shop attending to both.

The agency sees each individual on one designated day of the week, alphabetically according to last name. I guess that makes a certain amount of sense for the employment office in that it might expedite the agency's recordkeeping. But it certainly is not expeditious if you'd like to be the earliest bird to jump on a new job opening.

Being a vet, I was assigned a "counselor" from the agency's Veteran Employment Program. "No work is available for your skills at this time. We will contact you as soon as something comes up. In the meantime just stop by periodically and touch base. Hang in there, buddy; something will come up."

Filling up with skepticism— make that *cynicism*—I asked, "How many vets have you found jobs for within the past month?"

"Well, not so many, actually. You have to understand: a significant proportion of former service personnel petitioning us for employment opportunities bring with them an experiential background comprised primarily of combat training, which obviously constitutes a meager frame of reference by which to procure civilian employment. It would enhance those individuals' abilities to transition into the mainstream economy if the military were to provide its personnel with specific skills developments in order to augment their occupational preparation prior to their release from active duty."

Voice On My Shoulder tapped me and whispered. *Oh, gag, Lewis. Hide bureaucratic incompetence behind a cloak of big words. Shields up, Captain!*

Aloud, my own voice said to My Counselor, "Well, Sir, it doesn't matter much whether the incompetent one is you, or the Army; you're all government workers."

Nothing had changed; they were playing the same old game they were ten years ago. Get work for a handful of ex-GIs and call it "positive action for America's veteran community," and spin the press releases so as to justify keeping all those intellectually challenged inepts on the government payroll.

When I returned to my parents' place, where Tina and I were "temporarily" staying while we sought our own housing, my dad greeted me. "How'd it go, Chuck?"

"Frustrating. Christ, the government is mired so deep in its own crap they all have brown eyes."

"Well, Son, you just hang in——"

"Arraugghh!" My maniacal howl interrupted my dad and he didn't even try to finish his platitude.

After partaking of my mother's fine table Tina settled me down to go over the Houses For Rent section in the newspaper, all the while assuring me that everything was going to work out for us. I don't know how she did it, but she sure had a way of mellowing me out. "You have to admit, Chuck, that the employment people must do *something* right; sometimes they do find work for people. They just don't know how to look through a veteran's glasses."

The way my wife handled stress and pressure ... with her for an anchor and lifeline, then yes, everything was going to work out. Damn, how I loved her.

I must have gone through every piece of paper I owned a dozen times, making sure I had every document the Veterans Administration could possibly need. First and foremost was my DD-214, the most important paper a discharged serviceman receives. Without the 214, there can be no school, no VA home loan, no disability compensation, no medical benefits. Nothing.

Early, early Monday morning I mounted up my Mustang and rode into Seattle. I wanted to be there to open up shop—mostly because I hate waiting in lines. I was the second man through the door. The first thing I did was wait. The staff needed to finish their coffee and box of Dunkin Donuts Six Varieties, I guess.

After a half hour I got out my honey-coated voice and approached the front desk. "I see you're encountering a little unexpected delay. I was thinking I could save your staff some time and lighten the workload if you could give me my papers to fill out now, while I await my turn."

"Sorry, sir. Go ahead and be seated and someone will be with you shortly."

Three-quarters of an hour after the office opened for business, I became the first client to be called for interview.

The fellow who lives in me, whom I call Voice On My Shoulder, chuckled. *Let's see. At an average of thirteen dollars an hour times three-quarters of an hour times the number of employees in the office times the number of working days per year, how much do taxpayers pay the VA to dunk donuts?*

The VA service rep first wanted to see my documents. Yes, I was duly discharged and yes, I had permanent files with the Army.

"Now, Mr. Lewis, let's take care of the proper paperwork appropriate for each VA service or benefit you wish to apply for."

"I want to go to school."

He took out the sheaf of "go to school" forms and started firing questions.

"Your educational goals?"

"I haven't decided. I've been in The Other World Of The Military so long I don't even know what all the careers are these days. I know I want to train for a career, but I need just a tiny bit of time to find out what's out there."

"Have you enrolled or been accepted at a local college?"

"I have been out of the Army for a sum total of 120 hours. No, I haven't yet chosen a college. Besides, the next term won't start for two, three months. I figured that gave me a little time to avoid a hasty decision about the rest of my life."

"You haven't much information for us to go on."

"It seemed to me like the first step was to find out for sure that the VA was going to help me through school. Doesn't make sense to start classes and then find out I can't get GI educational benefits."

I asked for the application forms for my Certificate of Eligibility, which I would need to buy a home in the future.

"That's assuming you'll have the finances to purchase one," the rep said, fixing his face into Fake Smile Number Six.

"That's what I'm here for."

I felt it beginning to seep out of this guy: arrogance with a fringe of disdain around it. It's a front people try putting up when they're a little slow, or maybe to mask their impatience. I reminded myself that all he does day in and day out is ask the same questions and get the same answers from us ignorant vets. He must get tired of the same old thing day after day. On the other hand, that's his job. And he does get some pretty damn good donut-dunkin' comp time.

"Moving on, Mr. Lewis. Have you any disabilities to claim?"

Ah! The question I've been waiting for! "Actually, yes. Foot injury and back injury from Vietnam wounds. Hearing loss. Crohn's disease contracted as a result of military service——"

"We have some papers for you to fill out. You can complete the form at home and return it by mail. In the meantime, the VA will procure your service medical records from the Army."

"I have a complete copy of my official medical records right here . . ." I began pulling papers from the fat file of documents I had with me.

"We can't use copies. We have to have the originals."

I could understand that. A veteran must prove that claimed disabilities are the result of his or her service duties. Quite often people try to obtain compensation for medical problems that have nothing to do with their military service.

My particular health and medical problems, however, were all one hundred percent related to and a direct result of my service. Tom, a medic friend in Germany, figured my disability rating would be at least sixty, possibly eighty percent, and Tina and I concurred with his calculation. My compensation, while it would not be enough to bring us up to poverty level, would enable Tina and me and our baby to at least survive until I was through school and established in a job.

Tina and Mom were still out running around when I arrived home shortly after noon. I made coffee then settled down to peruse the endless supply of brochures the VA service rep gave me. Information about VA home loans, all the VA benefits and deadlines for filing, an explanation of the educational program. All dry reading, but all informative.

There was also a listing of college courses and degree programs. As I studied the blurbs I scratched out the programs I had no interest in and made my own list of those I thought I would like and do well in. That way, when Tina went over the programs with me later on, I would already have things narrowed down.

Then I started filling out the form for my disability claim. I pulled out all my military medical records so I would have all the information correct; I did not want any foul-ups that Tom the medic once told me were practically *modus operendi.*

I was in another flair-up stage of Crohn's disease, which certainly made it easy for me to know what to complain about on the forms for the physical. I was in a noticeable amount of lower abdominal pain, and people stared when I grabbed my side as a strong contraction hit me.

The form said *State the problem for which you wish to claim benefits. List only symptoms; do not state specific diagnosis.*

I thought it strange the VA didn't want to know what I actually *had*. I mean, if you just say you have a stomach ache, who's to know whether it's from appendicitis, cancer, labor pains, food gone bad, or too much chocolate cake? "Stomach ache" is a symptom, all right, but it doesn't say whether you'll be fine in the morning, or dead next week.

I noted my foot and back problems and my hearing loss and added the notation," Previous diagnosis of Crohn's Disease or some other form of colitis." That would give the examining MD a starting point. I also noted my daily bouts of diarrhea. The fact of my life now was the ever-present chance of embarrassment in public. The first thing I did when I went anywhere was to find out where the closest restroom was, and I didn't go any place that didn't have one. My weight bounced between 160 and 190, sometimes overnight, it seemed. When I got up each morning I never knew whether to pull on the size thirty-two jeans or the thirty-eights.

Tina came home radiant with excitement and smiling like the cat that swallowed the canary, and talking sixty per.

"I talked to a priest about joining that church—you know, that one we drove by and commented about how it looked so nice for an older building—and he got me all set up with a government-sponsored program that will provide free prenatal care and a free delivery—get that, *free delivery*?—and they even pay the hospital bills and I can't believe our good luck."

I grabbed my wife around the waist, picked her up and whirled her around. Then I gave her a long hug. I let her think the hug was because I loved her so much, but it really was because I had to collect my emotions. I had been terrified about the major league expense of having a baby, and us with no insurance.

"God, Hon," I said when I trusted my voice. "Who says it doesn't pay to go to church?"

2

The first thing we did to show we were now citizens of The Great State Of Washington was . . . we bought fishing licenses. Which wasn't at all frivolous, if you think about it, because the next important thing on my agenda was choosing a community college. Community colleges like you better if you're a tax-paying resident; my license and salmon tags were part of my documents of residency.

From the many brochures and college catalogs, I narrowed my choice to two favorites. I discovered that Ft. Steillacoom Community College had one of the Northwest's best veterinary assistant's programs, and the idea of working with animals appealed to me. Besides, I prefer being around animals over most people I know. Yes, I firmly resolved, that was what I would enjoy doing for the rest of my working life. So FSCC was the school I visited first.

The campus was impressive, the helpful people in its offices even more so. Of course I realized their cordiality was part sales pitch: I was the prospective new student ready to have my gray matter stimulated with higher learning, and in return they get my money. It's the American Way; nothing is free.

My other choice, Green River Community College in Auburn, had essentially the same curriculum as Ft. Steillacoom, except that Green River didn't offer veterinary courses. But it wouldn't make much difference which school I went to the first year because each required the same basic classes.

My bottomline consideration of the moment was that I wanted to be present at my baby's birth. Green River was twenty miles from Tina's hospital; Ft. Steillacoom was thirty-five.

It wasn't until I was filling out my enrollment application at GRCC that I was told about a break I hadn't counted on. Washington state reduces tuition for Vietnam vets. Maximum tuition for a full load of classes was (in 1981) $84 per quarter. Plus books, fees, parking, and the like; but any way you added it up it was an educational bargain.

With Tina's delivery and medical care arranged for and my enrolling at GRCC, we felt we were beginning to put the pieces in place for our financial future. We had our plan outlined:

... We would accept Mom and Dad's invitation to stay with them until my veteran's benefits commenced.

... Tina would go to work part time after she had the baby. We would coordinate our schedules to share child care. That agreement was a condition of my getting out of the Army. I really counted on her doing her part.

... My working while attending school was out of the question. School was never a snap for me; I had to work at studenthood. Farther along in my veterinarian course I would take an internship, but not the first year. Our income would consist of my VA benefits and Tina's wages.

Of course, we didn't know precisely what kind of figures we were working with because I hadn't yet received any benefits. In fact, I had not heard from the VA since I left my "counselor's" office. God, they're slow. If we weren't so financially strapped, if I didn't so desperately need a settlement *right now,* it might be rather fun, I thought, to see if my claim would set a VA record for Slow.

In the middle of February we found a mobile home in Prairie Ridge, and our other car arrived from Germany. Now we had a home to go to and a car for each of us to go to it in.

The mobile was perfect for our immediate needs. It was a fourteen-by-seventy with a large tip-out and —get this!—a fireplace in the living room. That was a big bonus feature to me; I'm partial to fireplaces. It cost more than I really wanted to commit, not knowing what our income would be; but we pledged to be very frugal until I got my disability award.

The first of March, 1981 we assumed occupancy of our new home and days later our household goods arrived from Germany. We now had a house full of stuff, I began receiving my unemployment compensation, I started school; and all the necessary paperwork, processes, protocols, and procedures had been initiated with the VA. Life was flowing along smoothly.

The VA finally scheduled my physical exam for the disability compensation award. Knowing it would be slated as it was during the school term, I deliberately took a light class load. If the physical was done properly and completely I would have a complete G.I. series, and that always laid me up for a few days; the Crohn's made it extremely painful to pass the barium. So taking fewer classes gave me a better whack at catching up after recuperating from my physical.

Tina accompanied me to the VA Medical Center in Seattle. She knew that after the exam I would be in no shape to drive; the X-ray procedure always caused me so much pain I could never drive myself home.

As soon as I checked in I was handed a form to fill out. It seemed like the same one I filled out to apply for the medical disability. Now why the hell can't they just pull my file? Don't they ever *read* those hundreds of thousands of fill-in-the-blanks questions you answer? Oh, well, this is not a good time to annoy any bureaucrats, so I started filling the blanks.

I was still confused about the item about "present complaint." All they wanted was the symptoms. I basically copied it just the way the Army doctors wrote it up in my service record, figuring that would be the most help to the VA doc.

> Item 17. Present Complaint (symptoms only, not diagnosis)
>
> 1. Lack of movement & pain of (R) foot after prolonged walking/standing
>
> 2. Low back pain after prolonged physical activity. (i.e. Lifting, walking, sitting; running is impossible; restricted movement.
>
> 3. Low abdominal pain accompanied by blood in stools (colitis)
>
> 4. Distinguished loss of hearing

Twenty minutes later the doctor called me in. After the introduction and the How do you do, the great inquisition began.

"How are we feeling today?"

"I'm pretty well considering the circumstances."

I did not realize it then, but as I sure learned later, the politely spoken "How do you feel today?" is a loaded question. If you answer in any affirmatives the doctor takes it that you are in better condition than you may really be. Usually "How are you?" ... "Fine" is a greeting, a hello, nothing more or less. When that exchange involves a VA doctor, though, he assumes your complaint for disability is not as serious as it actually is. You have set yourself up for a fall. From that point on you will not convince the doctor you have a serious problem, and he will play down the real level of your problem.

The doctor sat back and perused my military records, comparing them with my claim for disability. Then he began to quiz me.

"How's your foot injury?"

"It's coming along pretty well. It gives me difficulty only now and then."

"What kind of difficulty do you have? How did you receive the injury?"

"My foot was crushed between two deuce and a half trucks in an incident in Vietnam. Pains shoot through my foot and up my leg. When I have a day of standing and walking the spasms increase, and the big toe swells and becomes tender."

"Can you identify one specific incident that may have caused your back problems?"

"It might have happened on any number of occasions, or an accumulation of traumas. It could have occurred during a parachute jump. Or one or some of the several times I was shot down when I was a door gunner. I remember hitting hard a couple of the times our chopper went down. A sudden drop straight down, and the impact while sitting on a steel plate that does not absorb shock is probably as good a way as any to injure a person's back." I doubted this guy had any sense of irony or humor at all, but—for my own relief and amusement, mostly—I added, "I am proof that it's not the fall that gets ya, it's that sudden stop at the end."

The doctor pressed on. "You can't nail down one specific point of injury?"

"I could probably nail down half a dozen bumps, shocks, and owies. A couple of Army doctors thought the back problem relates to the crushed foot. One doc thought it was because my hips are out of alignment; the misalignment is due to one leg being about three-quarters of an inch shorter than the other."

The doc inhaled to start another sentence, but I hastily continued on before he squelched my chance to say all I wanted to tell him.

"What I am sure of is that my back has a habit of seizing up and locking, with every attached muscle drawing up so tightly that any attempt to move causes excruciating pain. I'm not trained in anatomy or medicine, so I do not understand what sets off freezing-up of muscles."

I am well aware that the medical profession has found the reason for back problems to be one of the most difficult things to pinpoint and diagnose, and that a lot of soldiers and sailors use "backache" as a foolproof excuse to malinger. Maybe I was the one-in-four arbitrarily selected to be turned down, a chosen one predestined to pay the price for other people's cheating. On the other hand, I was beginning to get resentful. If trained physicians can't figure out why a man's back won't work, how the hell did they expect me to?

The doctor moved on to the next point. "How much loud noise were you exposed to, and how often?"

"I was a weapons specialist. I spent a very great deal of time firing many sorts of weapons and using demolitions to blow things up. During an attack in Nam a rocket hit the top of my bunker, and that rang my chimes for about a week. Exposure to all the pyrotechnics used in assorted field training exercises took a toll as well. I was assigned to Mech Infantry and that means dealing with tanks and personnel carriers—vehicles which are not known for being quiet. I spent time as a doorgunner, and there's nothing like the high-pitched scream of that transmission right behind your head."

There was a long history of hearing tests in my official records to support that part of my claim.

Now the doc got to the meat of my disability claim, the Crohn's disease issue, only he wouldn't call it that. "How long have you had this digestive problem?" he asked.

"Since 1979. I thought at first I was having minor episodes of dysentery or some such tropical malady. I spent most of my time in the field, where cuisine was not served under not the most sanitary conditions, so at first that seemed a reasonable cause for the problem. Although it seemed awfully persistent for what you'd call 'a passing problem,' I thought I could control it on my own. I always had an aversion to going on sick call. And that is why the condition is not written up on my records early on.

"The pain grew steadily worse, then on New Years Eve of 1979 it was so bad I couldn't move. My wife and a neighbor literally carried me to the car. By the time the hospital got around to seeing me it was New Years Day of 1980. I spent thirty days in the hospital, bouncing around between the surgeon's knife and the internist, who, thank God, won out."

I explained how the internist was pretty sure I had Crohn's disease, and I produced a letter from the doctor which said so. I also showed the VA doc some additional medical files I copied from my records prior to my discharge.

"How are you doing now since your discharge?"

"The sudden attacks of diarrhea and the lack of bowel control are still a major problem, a source of constant aggravation. I am having difficulty dealing with the accompanying pain. Sometimes the pain is so unbearable that if I happen to be standing when it hits, it takes my legs right out from under me. I am talking about some totally awesome pain threshold here, Doctor."

"What medication are you taking for pain? For diarrhea?"

"Nothing, because I don't have access to a doctor right now; that is why I am here. I don't remember what the doctors in Germany had me taking."

"How many flare-ups have you had since you got out of the Army?"

"Three major episodes in just over two months. I basically treated myself. No solid food. When I am doing okay I eat only once a day, that being supper, and I eat at home where the facility is close. It's not the best way to handle the situation but it works for me."

I explained that ever since the problem started back in '79 I was always in some degree of lower abdominal pain; whether it was slight or massive it is always there. It was simply a daily fact of life, as is the diarrhea.

"How many trips to the toilet per day?"

"It's directly proportional to the number of times I eat. I've learned to get along with only one meal a day, with an average of four to six, ah, rest stops. If I eat three meals it's ten to fifteen trips—which leaves very little time for anything else. So I only eat supper, and only at home."

I made a point to explain to him my total lack of bowel control. When the urge strikes there is no waiting around. I am talking about being within a few steps of a toilet, not a run from the back yard; but then, with the cramps and pain, running is not possible, anyway.

To make the case for my disability claim perfectly, abundantly clear, I added, "This is by far and without exception the most serious problem I have to deal with. What I really fear is that it's so serious it will interfere with my employability."

The doc weighed and measured me, then asked me to strip to my skivvies. He checked the flexibility of my back and measured my legs—presumably to see if one leg was shorter.

Then I lay on the table and he started applying pressure to my abdomen—a little vigorously, I thought. When he pressed hard on the lower right quadrant, I came right off the table and almost went through the ceiling.

"Did that hurt?" he asked innocently.

"No, I always go from horizontal into orbit for no reason." *Hell yes it hurt, you damn fool.*

He instructed me back on the table and he did it *again*, I guess to be sure he was right the first time. Then he twisted my bum foot and tried to bend toes that didn't bend because the joints had been fused. Then he told me I could get dressed and go to the lab for x-rays and a hearing test.

"Yeah," I mumbled, rubbing my foot. "Assuming I can walk."

I opted for the hearing test first because it didn't involve stripping, prodding, or pain. It was the standard hearing test I've had so often. It took no time at all.

At the x-ray lab I waited around the prescribed forty minutes, then was called in for my photo session.

"Well," I told Tina on the drive home, "so much for the Veterans Administration Disability Physical. The only x-rays taken were two shots of my foot, a couple of my back, and the required chest x-ray."

"How about the Crohn's?" she asked.

"That's what surprised me most. There was no lab work whatsoever, no work-up for the Crohn's disease at all. No upper and lower G.I. series."

"So they don't know any more than the Army doctors did? Which is nothing?" Tina's brow furrowed. "How can the VA verify your claim without the tests?"

"Maybe the Army records are good enough for them to make a decision," I said. "I certainly wasn't about to tell this guy how to run a physical; who am I to tell a doctor how to do his job? Besides," I grinned, "I definitely was not looking forward to being laid up for the next two or three days while I recovered from those damn barium-filled tests."

"When are we going to get your money?"

The money of course was the bottom line, but Tina's bluntness and her tone made it sound so ... mercenary.

"They told me not to expect any information for sixty to ninety days." I reached over and patted my wife's thigh. "Just think, Hon, in three months I'll have a quarter of college, a child, and an income that'll scrape us by. God bless America."

3

With the hassle of the physical behind me, it was a matter of waiting to hear from the VA. But I had plenty to do without just sitting around stewing.

Tina was starting to show, and we were into reading the books and articles on babies and parenting.

And I got serious about being a student. I hummed along in all my classes except algebra. I couldn't pass an exam if my life depended on it, regardless of how hard I studied.

After failing the mid-term I figured I was overdue for a private session with the professor. "I'm trying to make sense of it," I said. "I can't see why A over B equals C; it simply does not register with me."

"Well, Chuck, you aren't exactly destined to be a math major, so why don't you quit trying to get things to make sense. Just take my word for it that the mathematical system works. Follow the formulas, do as I say, and don't try to analyze *why* it works."

I'll be damned, he was right. I applied what he said and made straight A's the second half of the term, ended up with a C-plus. Damn, was I ever proud of myself. First time I ever got even a passing grade in algebra.

Tina, whether she planned it or not, did her part to keep me occupied as well. She was one of those women who, even though she had a smooth pregnancy, continuously went into false labor. Throughout April, we made the weekly mad dash to the hospital, one, two, three times a week. I'd go to class half asleep from late-night false-alarm runs.

On Saturday, May 2, 1981, we borrowed a friend's boat and spent the day fishing on Puget Sound. While she was doing the dishes that evening, Tina's water broke.

"This is no false alarm," she said, and we were both laughing because we were so happy.

"I've been in labor since we got off the boat, but I had no intention of telling you that before supper," she said as we raced for Seattle. "They won't let me eat once I get to the hospital, you know, and I don't want to do all that work on an empty stomach."

"Hon, I'd've put you on that boat long ago if I'd've known it would get this over with."

Mom and Dad met us at the hospital. We waited together.

Just after midnight Tina was moved from Labor to Delivery. The doctor and his team were nice and slow and leisurely, but Tina wasn't. They were still getting things ready when all of a sudden I had my hands full of baby daughter.

"Will you guys speed things up," I ordered the room full of scrubs who said their name was We Are Your Professional Team. "I don't know what to do with this handful of baby." At one in the morning of May third, Andrea Lewis bounced into her daddy's hands more literally than she will ever understand.

I stayed with my family until they were taken to their rooms. *My family—mother, father, baby. Oh, God, we are a full-fledged family.* Mom and Dad and I went out to breakfast, then I went home and made all the obligatory calls to the rest of the family.

Man, was I fried when I got to class the next morning! By the time I got to Oral Communication I was exhausted, and anxious to get it over with so I could get to the hospital to see my family. Not so fast, Lewis, not until you take time off to celebrate. A couple of students bought champagne and there we were, partying with alcohol in a public school. Our professor really put his neck on the limb that day. I guess he could have been fired, the rest of us suspended or expelled; but I think it's okay to pull one over on the establishment once in a while.

I finished my first term at college with an A, a B, and two C's—and a new baby. I looked forward to the next term; I was no longer a New Freshman.

It had been over three months and I still had heard nothing from the VA. I enrolled for summer term to keep my benefits flowing. The added expense of a new family member continued to build, and still nothing about a settlement from the VA. Adding to that, Tina's younger sister came to stay with us and go to school. She attended a beautician school in Auburn, and while her parents paid her school expenses, I was stuck with the rest of her support. She was a help to Tina but it added to our living expenses.

On August 6, 1981 I finally received the letter of decision from the VA.

> Your claim for Disability Compensation has been approved as follows:
>
> | MONTHLY RATE | EFFECTIVE DATE |
> |---|---|
> | $275 | 1-15-81 |
> | $289 | 5-03-81 |
>
> You will be promptly notified of additional scheduled changes in your award beyond the period shown above.
>
> Service connection has been established for:
>
> | | |
> |---|---|
> | RESIDUALS OF FOOT INJURY, RIGHT | 20% |
> | SACROILIAC CONDITION | 20% |
> | IMPAIRED HEARING | 0% |
> | COMBINED | 40% |
>
> The combined evaluation is not determined by adding the percentage of your disabilities as shown but is computed by using a combined rating table.
>
> Service connection is not established for:
>
> TINITUS
> CONDITION OF DIGESTIVE SYSTEM
>
> Included are additional benefits for your spouse and children.
> Any change in the number or status of your dependents must be reported promptly to the VA.

THANK YOU,

VETERANS ADMINISTRATION

This decision totally denied me any benefits for Crohn's Disease. It didn't even recognize its presence. I was dumbfounded by this rating. It was insane. I had explained everything in detail, as carefully and thoroughly as I could. How could they justify denying this, which they circumvent and minimize by referring to it as a "condition of the digestive system"? They had my Army medical records. They had a mass of additional information I provided to ensure all the bases were covered.

The other decisions are fair, but I can not live with this. I did my homework. I know this disease is going to mess up my life even more than it is. If I don't get this changed, the rest of my life will be all but ruined.

I called the VA office to try to find out the reason for the decision.

"You'll have to file for a Statement of Case," said an impersonal voice.

The tone of the voice said, "Sigh. Here we go again."

"Then you will have to file an appeal," said the voice. "We'll send the form for you to request the Statement of Case."

Reason for the decision? They have no reason.

I started to investigate — *they* certainly aren't going to — and discovered that the information the VA used in determining my case was absolutely bogus.

Document: "Compensation & Pension Evaluation Summary." Date: March 27, 1981. "Physical examination ref Rectal Hemoccult Negative Stool."

According to that, I was tested for blood in my stools or rectum and none was found.

What a crock; I was never given such a test. I would remember a rectal exam if I had one!

What is going on here? Clearly this was nothing but a bold faced lie.

But more good stuff was yet to come.

Document: "Rating Decision." Date: July 21, 1981. "Veteran denied having blood in stool or subsequent pain since Nov. 1980. Colitis was not found on V.A.E."

Now wait a goddamned minute here! On my request for a physical I specifically stated in writing that I had pain and bleeding, and the problem was getting worse. And let's not forget: my official Army medical records note I was treated for pain and bleeding in December 1980.

So there I had it: Two pages of description and detail in my file reduced to a two-line lie. No wonder there was no signature on the letter.

I simply could not figure any justification for my denial of claim, a denial based on un-facts and misconclusions. I had done everything but draw the doctor a picture of my problem. Surely it's some kind of clerical error, I reasoned. The United States Government would not deliberately go out of its way to deny an individual the benefits given him by law. That's it; there has to be a mistake somewhere.

A couple of other vets were in my college classes. I hailed them down to talk about it.

"Whatta fun day for the ol' VA!" Ralph chanted.

"Yeah, you bet. They screwed another vet!" Max rapped.

"Hey, we know a whole truckload of stories about vets being ripped out of their benefits," said Ralph.

"The Veterans Administration couldn't care less about the veterans they are supposed to be serving," said Max. "No reason for you to expect anything from them, either."

To me people who yelled rip-off were just sneaks who tried to get more than they had coming to them, and when they couldn't they cried foul. "After all, Max, I do have a bonafide problem and it's doomed to get progressively worse. If it isn't treated, I'll ultimately end up with surgical removal of my intestines."

"You going to request an appeal?" Ralph asked.

"You bet your sweet ass I am. And I'll go loaded with information and back-up documents. But I shouldn't have to. I just simply do not understand how they could deny me my entitlements based on information they didn't have. Or how they took what they did have and ass-back it. Or how that guy could sit there in his office and tell me my exam was complete and now come back on me and tell me I didn't have enough lab work."

Just talking about it, I was beginning worry myself. "If this case does end up being long and strung out, then the lack of lab work as evidence could really hurt my case, couldn't it?"

Max nodded soberly. "You could definitely be in a world of shit if that happens."

Even with the award I got, combined with my unemployment — a total $564 a month — Tina and I were over our heads financially. Tina pretended to be surprised we were broke. She was defensive about the extravagances she indulged herself; she acted hurt when I mentioned that her sister's keep was setting us back. She refused to grasp the concepts of needs versus wants and she had no understanding of prioritizing. Pinched and crunched, we gave up our mobile home and moved back in with my family. "Just until I find some work and a cheaper place to live," I told Dad.

As it turned out, I was the only one who ended up living there. Tina's sister went back to her parents' place in New York, and Tina and Andrea and went with her.

I quit school and went out looking for work. No luck of any kind.

Funny how the cards change, practically overnight. Two months ago ... a new family, college, a ton of optimism. Today ... all crumbled to hell. I working up a good belligerence toward the VA, laying the blame on them for screwing up my life. Feeling charity toward none and malice toward all, I went to the regional office to file my appeal.

4

The receptionist asked if I intended to use a service representative from one of the local veterans organizations. At first I was skeptical about that because I never had a good experience with such groups. They were there to look out for the vets from World War Two and Korea; like most of Americana, the Organization Men didn't consider us Vietnam vets to be true-definition veterans. On the other hand, I realized I would need the help of someone who knew how the system worked (or get *around* the workings). I wanted a speedy resolution to this obvious error, and in the end I decided the service reps should be the most in-the-know ones to help me.

So I went downstairs to see the representative of Disabled American Veterans (DAV.).

The first thing he did was hit me up for a ten dollar membership fee.

"If you are a member we can offer so much more help to you," was the rep's subtle hint.

Same-old MO. Nothing has changed in the past fifteen years. But you need all the support you can get. Oh, well, at least you'll get a magazine subscription. Intimidation works, Voice. I forked over the ten.

The rep, a nice enough dude named Sam, reassured me. "Your case is pretty cut and dried, no sweat."

I gave Sam all the information he needed. "Plus more to come," I said. "I have additional information at home, and I'll be collecting more." Then I signed over a power of attorney so he could act on my behalf.

Then Sam gave me the drill about how to conduct myself before doctors and hearing boards.

"Look as bad as is reasonably possible, because they will use your outward appearance and demeanor against you. Do not admit you are feeling well—and for God's sake, when they say 'How are you?' don't say, 'Fine.' If you're disabled, you see, you are *not* fine and don't say you are."

Sam asked me how I was getting along otherwise. I explained about my college work and the job search.

"Well, you're certainly pulling your own bootstraps," Sam said. "Not sitting around waiting for freebies to be handed out or anything like that. Let's get you set up with VA's Vocational Rehabilitation Department." He tapped my award letter on his desk. "You needed to be rated at least thirty percent disability to qualify for VA Rehab, and you already have a forty percent. You're entitled to rehab, Mr. Lewis, but you should have gotten yourself into the program sooner."

"Never heard of the program. The VA didn't seem to want to share that little tidbit about a goody vets are entitled to."

Sam sent me to Voc Rehab, and the first thing they did was (ta-daahh): give me . . .

. . . more forms to fill out.

Surprise, surprise!

First, I had to be rated at "30 percent disability or more" — No problem there — and be judged as having "non-civilian-related skills from the military."

In other words, there is no suitable civilian counterpart to the position of Infantryman in the Army.

What a crock. Especially for one who has attained a position of leadership and authority in the Infantry. Infantry NCOs are experienced leaders. They manage personnel and material. They are accountable and responsible for timely and accurate filing of reports and surveys. They do what thousands of civilian managers and CEOs do every day.

As a platoon sergeant I was responsible for millions of dollars worth of equipment; for supervising upwards of sixty-five men, solely accountable and responsible for their conduct, job performance, training and development; for maintaining accurate records and reports; and for conducting a myriad of missions all the while I was doing everything else. I think I have a grasp of what management is about, and my grasp comes from the best educational program of all: experience.

Above all, military people have a more detailed understanding of the concept of *Loyalty* than most of their civilian counterparts — civilian-world businessmen and bureaucrats and social workers, milk-toast sissies who call themselves managers but who start looking for Stress Support Groups if they have more than a couple of tasks at a time, then refuse to accept full responsibility for their actions or conduct. Pass the buck. It isn't my fault; it's society's fault, or something my mother did when I was five months old, or politics, the national debt, the weather, bad schools, not enough law enforcement, God's will. No wonder our society is in the state it's in. Damn, what a waste of talent and human resources.

The secretary at Voc Rehab reviewed my paperwork and told me it was complete and in good order. "A rehab counselor will be in touch in a day or two and set up an appointment."

Why do we always have to make an appointment to come in and be told they'll call to make an appointment?

During this time my Crohn's suddenly went into overdrive. My guts killed me. My innards tied themselves in knots and little gremlins inside pulled the knots tighter. My basic habitat was the can. When I reached the outer threshold of agony, I dragged myself to the VA hospital for treatment, hoping I wouldn't have an accident in the car.

All I wanted was pain-relief medication. I absolutely did not want to be admitted as an inpatient; I didn't have time for that. That was wasted worry; the hospital wouldn't see me nor treat me.

"Sorry, Mr. Lewis. By policy, we can only treat veterans whose specific problem is diagnosed as service-connected," says the homely bat at the walk-in clinic.

What kind of shit is this? "Look, Misses. I am sick, in severe pain, and I am a veteran trying to see a doctor at the veterans hospital. I have no insurance because the VA is so slow with my claim, and I damn sure can't afford to go to a civilian doctor. I was always under the assumption that any destitute veteran could get medical care at a VA hospital." *Besides, this would serve as additional evidence for my appeal.*

"Sorry. I can not see where you qualify."

"Ma'am," I said to the bitch, "I know alcoholics who go to the VA hospital to dry out. You're saying a vet with a serious medical problem and no resources gets turned away?"

I cannot accept that alcoholism is a service connected disability. Or is it that these are World War Two and Korean vets, and they are somehow more credible vets than us Nam slobs, that a man's blood is more honorable when it's shed in a *declared* war?

I could not afford to ire this crab, so I kept my tongue. Instead, I used my kind and diplomatic voice to explain that I was still seeking official recognition that my illness was indeed service connected, that an error in my physical was under appeal.

"Fine. When it is declared service connected we will be happy to treat you. In the meantime you'll have to go elsewhere as a welfare case."

I must have been struck dumb and numb because after a silence she dismissed me with, "I'm sorry, Mr. Lewis, but we have to deal with regulations due to budget restrictions."

"Damn, lady, nobody hollered budget restrictions when I was asked to do some shit-work for this country, and I don't accept that as a reason now." I no longer felt the need to be diplomatic.

I almost wished I'd crapped my pants while I stood in that nurse's territory.

I went back home in the same pain I left in.

I planted myself in bed, then sent my mom to the store for the items I needed to maintain myself a few days on a diet of clear liquids. The key to relief with Chron's Disease is to relax the digestive system and drink ample fluids to prevent dehydration, which is a serious side effect. The condition is much better controlled with hospitalization, but when you are without, you make due with what you have. But I sure could have made do a lot better if I had something for the pain.

Mom was about to go crazy with worry. "Go to my doctor," she urged.

Hell, I can't pay her doctor, and she really can't afford it, either. So I tried to ease her worry by assuring her this is business-as-usual for the disease. "In another day or two it will start to level off so I can join life again. Don't worry about me, Mom. I'm learning to deal with it." *Another ten days is more like it, but I'm not going to worry her with that.*

VA Voc Rehab called to announce an appointment the coming week. I hoped my current flare-up would be stable enough by then to get myself to the office.

Fortunately for me, it was. I arrived right on time and was ushered right in. A good omen, please God, for better things to come.

It's too bad the VA doesn't have more counselors like Dan Southerland.

We introduced ourselves. When Dan offered the usual "How are you?"— he got the story of my non-treatment at the VA hospital.

"Oh for God's sake!" Dan slammed his fist onto his desktop with such momentum it brought him halfway to his feet. "You had already applied for voc rehab, it says so right here." Then, more calmly, "As of this moment you *are* in voc rehab, and you are therefore eligible for any medical treatment at any VA hospital, guaranteed, and don't let any of those self-serving, gold-bricking bureaucrats try to tell you otherwise."

The reason I would be eligible, Dan explained, is that the VA has decreed that its vocational rehabilitation program *will* succeed, and they will not allow a student to use his or her medical problems as an excuse for failure. Therefore, they take care of the student.

"As your counselor, Mr. Lewis, and as the guy the buck stops at, I won't accept any excuses for any problems at school."

"The buck stops on your desk? I admire that. I like that, sir. We can work together."

We began discussing my career goals and the school program that would get me there. I told him of my decision to complete the Veterinary Assistant program.

I was immediately shot right out of the saddle.

"No veterinary training," he said firmly. "It requires lifting and manhandling large animals. That would cause further problems with your back injuries."

We debated the point, but I was forced to see the light. "I see your point is based on responsible common sense, Mr. Southerland, but damn, I wanted to work with animals!"

The only other option I had even considered was drafting. I enjoyed it in high school. I took a couple of correspondence courses in drafting when I was stationed in Germany.

"Green River College—where, I note, you have already attended—has one of the best drafting programs in the whole Northwest."

So it was written. I will get an Associate Degree in Drafting Technology.

Dan then explained the rules of the game. They were quite simple, and to me, fair and eminently doable.

—I would go to school and do well, no excuses.

—All my expenses—tuition, books, all supplies—would be paid for by the VA.

—I would receive the equivalent of GI Bill education benefits, along with disability compensation, to cover my living expenses. That gave me about eight hundred dollars a month, plus what was left of my unemployment comp.

Fall term had already started, so I would begin my new course in winter quarter, starting January 3.

Tina and little Andrea came back from New York and we got a place in Kent and made do with what we had. But I firmly believed that what we had would soon be added unto. I held that belief as I anticipated the upcoming re-evaluation of my claim for Crohn's Disease.

5

The Veterans Administration

December 2, 1982

Dear Mr. Lewis:

Veterans Administration records show that you have the following service-connected disability(ies):

DISABILITY	PERCENT
RESIDUALS OF FOOT INJURY	20
SACROILIAC CONDITION	20
IMPAIRED HEARING	0

Your combined rating is 40 percent.

You are awarded compensation of $324.00 per month.

Sincerely yours

"What in hell is this?" I raged to Tina. "This is exactly the same as it was before — a denial of benefits. I get another thirty-five a month — exactly the amount of the annual cost of living raise. What IS this?"

"Now, Honey," Tina soothed. "I'm sure it's just a clerical mistake, maybe a typo or something. Why don't you call that Disabled American what's-his-face and get it straightened out."

"Christalmighty, disabled is right!" I stormed, reaching for the phone.

"What's the deal with my new evaluation for Chron's Disease?" I asked Sam, my Disabled Representative at DAV. "What happened to my appeal?"

"Your request to correlate Chron's Disease to military service received negative response," Sam answered in stiff, elitist bureaucrappese.

"How could this happen? How did they arrive at this decision? Christ Almighty, what has been going on? And what information did they use to arrive at this stupid outrageous to-hell-with-you decision?"

"Does the judgment dissatisfy you, Mr. Lewis?"

Now what kind of asinine, pea-brained, moronic question was that? Bureaucratic sweet-and-light cop-out, of course. "Dissatisfied? Sam, Mr. Representative, I am thoroughly pissed. Now tell me, how did they arrive at this decision?"

"From the information from the original physical."

"There *was* no physical. There was no test. I mean, to hell with it all, that test — that they did *not* give me — was to be the very basis of my case. How hard is it to figure out that I was not tested properly the first time around, and you can not base an objective decision on nonexistent information. Gods, Sam, you knew that. That was what you were supposed to represent me on."

Silence.

"So, Mr. Sam, tell me. What happened to what was called my 'opportunity to present the new evidence'?"

Sam's tone took on that stubborn defensiveness people assume when they're confronted and they know they're wrong. "It was determined that such information was not necessary, and an adequate decision could be made without it," he simpered.

"Wait a damn minute here. Who the hell made that decision? I have the right to present any and all data and information pertinent to my case. Which I did. Reams of it. Which *'they,'* the infinite wise ones, ignored. What happened to due process?"

"Mr. Lewis, all I can say is the decision has been made, and if you choose to, you can file an appeal to the Board of Veterans Appeals."

"Okay. Now explain to me just what the hell that is, and what can they do for me?"

"The Board of Veterans Appeals is the high court set up by the Veterans Administration to hear cases of those who feel they have been treated wrong or have had their cases mishandled. You can have your hearing here at the Regional Office of the VA, or you can have it at National Office in Washington, D.C. In most cases the hearing is conducted locally, the transcripts forwarded to Washington for the final decision."

Oh groan. More formalese. Separate yourself from all possible real-person humanness. Well, I figured, effete-speak from him calls for pedestrian talk from me. "So how in hell do I initiate this action?" I barked.

"Well," Sam said, retaining his grease-slick smooth tone, "I can let the VA know your intentions, and they will issue a Statement of Case. You must follow up with your request for a hearing. Now I should remind you: this is a time consuming process, especially if you elect to carry your case to Washington."

"Let me get this straight, Sam. I notify the VA that I have intentions, then file an intent, then file a request to carry out my intent?"

"That is the protocol."

I poured myself a cup of five-hours-old coffee that was so awful it was perfect for my mood. "This is really terrific." I was really spewing to myself but Tina was in earshot so I suppose I was talking to her. "My case is being mishandled from the get-go, and all they do is stick me with a mess of red tape that will take God only knows how long to untangle. I can not, *not* understand how this could get so fucked up. All the VA had to do was spend a buck for a couple of lab tests and x-rays and all knowledge would be known. Jesus, am I asking for the impossible to think the VA could just handle this case?"

Tina moved behind me and rubbed the knots on my shoulders. "They said you'd get a hearing," she said softly.

"Yeah. Said. Assuming I do get one within the next six months, I'll be trying to prove what took place a year and a half in the past. With no medical tests to back me up for that period."

I let Tina's fingers do their work but I wasn't soothed. Nevertheless, I kept my mouth shut because there was no point in smashing her optimism; I needed for her to keep up her hope — our hope. I couldn't tell her about my haunting fear of trying to prove a point based on no legitimate back-up information from the VA. That trip to the hospital would have been great documentation, but the VA conveniently would not even see me.

This is not only nonsense; it is total incompetence.

Why do I get this feeling of being set up for a fall?

Tina and I had to move again because we couldn't afford the rent and expense of our place. Damn, I am tired of moving. If we had just another couple hundred bucks a month . . . We would have if the VA had handled my case properly in the first place.

We suffered through the Merry Holiday season, for what it was worth. I made sure Andrea had at least something for her first Christmas, and Tina and I exchanged a couple of little things; but getting into the season was difficult without finances.

My search for work was a total bust. It seemed that my twelve-plus years of service to the U.S. Government was a mistake. I swear it: As soon as a prospective employer found out I was so long in the Army, I was rejected. I went so far as to deny I spent those years in the service. That meant I had to fabricate a past—and that proved harder than telling the truth. I made crazy excuses as to why a former employer could not be contacted for a reference. I told one guy my old boss owned his own business ... that he died of a heart attack ... that I didn't know who took over the business.

The most destructive thing of all proved to be ... Tina. She had agreed — she promised — that as soon as she was recovered from childbirth she would go to work while I attended school. That was the condition *she* proposed to bribe me to leave the Army. Now she suddenly decided she wasn't going to work; she was going to college.

Here was a woman of great talent with great credentials in the media. She could operate cameras and switchboards, she could shoot commercials on location. Yet regardless of openings, she had no interest in applying or even inquiring.

I kept stumbling around trying to find work for myself. Anything that would make a buck. The best I could muster was an occasional odd construction jobs, a day or two now and then. Time I should have spent working I spent worrying about how we would manage with my lack of work.

Maybe my decision to get out of the Army was a mistake. I should have stayed in while this disease worsened and the Army had been forced to give me a medical retirement. Hell, I've heard of people getting medical retirements for stomach ulcers. What I had beat ulcers by a long shot, and I was tired of the VA insisting that what I had wasn't real. Dr. Hall suspected Crohn's Disease; all the other morons had to do was follow up. If they had done their job the VA wouldn't be denying me benefits.

Yes, I goofed up: I got out too soon, and I believed in the system.

Several times and in different ways, I reminded Tina of commitment she had made, and of her failure to honor it. She told her parents I was bugging her to go to work, and they let it be known that they thought of me as a useless bum. I explained to them of the agreement we made prior to my discharge, but they refused to accept it. In their eyes, their daughter was perfection incarnate.

Out of love for Tina, I dropped the issue. I did feel at least partly responsible for our misery ... hers, especially. And I really loved that lady. I was committed to my marriage, and the maintenance of my family was my responsibility and my priority.

I would discover new ways to stretch a dollar — just like thousands of other college students with families.

Winter term began and for once I was an actual scholar; it was as if I were a draftsman by nature. I was the first in my class to make a perfect score on a drawing. Each drawing was graded on accuracy and quality of line (pretty cut and dried), and neatness and quality of printing (the real killer). Printing was the hardest element to master, and few of us did.

This term I was truly intense in my studying and in pursuit of my degree. I had put in a term of BS-ing through the basics of getting back into the swing of school; now I flew through everything I could get.

I did, however, miss a substantial chunk of school because of Crohn's episodes, but I kept it controlled without going to that damn VA hospital. Twice, though, I went in for medication for lower-back pain. When I did, I pointedly mentioned the Crohn's, asking the doctor to enter it on my VA medical record and note the possibility of a relationship between Crohn's flare-ups and the back problem. Soon after a Crohn's episode the back gave out —something to do with the way I walked stooped over from the pain in my guts, I think. At least that is my (unproved) theory. If the docs cared, they could check out the theory ... maybe get themselves published in one of the revered medical journals.

I kept cruising along through school, quarter after quarter. I bought a drafting table so when I wasn't well enough to go to class I could keep up with the drawings ... keep up, heck; I did extra; by God, I had a creative knack. That table hit us up for about fifty smackers, which anyone familiar with drafting equipment will know is an outstanding buy. Tina took an interest in what I was doing, even helped me out at times.

My grades never faltered — solid three-point-three grade average, taking classes as fast as I could. Green River C-C considered ten credits a full time load and the VA required twelve. I clipped them off at eighteen a quarter and knocked out 24 in my final winter term. Damn, I was proud of myself. I never dreamed I could do this well in any school outside the military.

While I was cooking on four burners, Tina was growing irritable. Silly little picky things bugged her; but as I saw it, money was the root of all edginess. Our money problem revolved around Tina's spending habits, and then, suddenly, around the cost of rent.

Our apartment was perfect for us. Roomy. Only $250 a month.

Then the owner sold the building.

The new guy immediately raised the rent to four hundred and something a month. That was more than half my monthly income.

Christ, here we go again.

We tried to find some low income housing, but the waiting list was so long that I would be graduated from college by the time our name came up.

Back to my mom and dad's.

6

Tina picked the time of our move as her time to demand to start college.

"But our agreement was for you to work until I finished school, then *I* work and *you* start school," I reminded her. "If you had kept your part of the deal we wouldn't be bouncing around from one living quarters to another. We sure wouldn't be living at Mom and Dad's place right now."

Big mistake. Tina wocked out, straight off the deep end. I had never seen this woman raise so much hell with so much hostility, so bordering on insanity. *We can not afford a place to live, and I am expected to give her money to attend college?*

Tina remained adamant. She was going to school and start the drafting program and that was that. My bottom-line choice was either letting her go to school or losing her.

Maybe the school thing was just a symptom. Maybe she was frustrated because she felt she had no control over anything else right now, and as a student she would be in charge of at least that aspect of her life. All this moving around got to her. Living with her in-laws got to her. She was pissed that my VA case was so screwed up, and she was starting to blame me, hinting that it was I who was doing things wrong.

Tina's attitudes and actions took me by surprise. This was a side of her I had never seen; maybe it was never there until now. Though I knew it was a big mistake, I was in no mood to challenge her, and besides I was in love with her. Tina started college the fall of 1982.

Very soon I admitted to myself that my wife was really cut out for studenthood and draftsmanship. She grasped and understood the subject. Her drawings were meticulous and neat. She filled me with pride.

Besides that, the two of us going to school together — I got a real boot out of that.

"Chuck, you never cease to amaze me." Dan Southerland was still my counselor at VA voc rehab, and I was grateful for that. "Your transcript shows that you're about to graduate — a two-year Associate Degree in a year and a quarter. Amazing. With honors, already!"

"Barring any unforeseen problems," I cautioned him. I was getting to be a professional skeptic.

"Look, Chuck. With your aptitude, your interest, your focus — this is a calling, man. Why don't you consider going on and getting a full-fledged degree in engineering?"

"*Consider* it? That's been my ambition and goal since Day One. Except I can't afford it."

"Remember our first meeting? When I told you I would ride your be-hind so hard that failure was impossible? Well, I'm not riding you any more; I'm ready to forge ahead of you and make trail. It will only take a stroke of the pen to get you an exception to policy, Chuck."

I felt the grin going clear around my head. I reached over the desk and Dan and I clasped hands. "Then get out your pen."

My immediate problems blurred in the mist as I sharpened my focus on our future. With just a little more sacrifice we could tough it out for two more years. Damn ... me with a bachelor of science in engineering, Tina with an associate's in drafting ... both of us professionals in technological fields ... Andrea would have everything Tina and I never did ...

Oregon Institute of Technology accepted me into its engineering program. My course would begin in spring quarter in March. So during Christmas break Tina and I trekked the voyage to Klamath Falls to have a lookie. Awesomely beautiful country. Delightful community. And cutting edge, state-of-the-art, high-reputation school of engineering.

Many miles before arriving at K-Falls, I knew we were likely to find affordable housing. This was no Silicon Valley chip economy; it was agriculture, ranching, timber. A classified cruise through the local newspaper proved I was right: three, four bedroom houses rented for two-fifty to three hundred a month.

The only hurdle on the track was that I had just one week's time between finishing my finals at Green River C-C and starting at OIT. Well, I could certainly clear that low hurdle; all I need do is ... a-*hem* ... "engineer" a plan, everything in the right sequence—and all the time, of course, keeping up in my final quarter at GRCC.

I drafted my blueprint:

—Schedule a four-day block to go to K-Falls to find housing. We would need to have a place waiting to move into so I could start classes on time. VA rules required me to start immediately, without missing a beat.

—Tina could hold off a term, get the household established, find child care for Andrea.

—By mid-quarter (my final term at GRCC), have all forms and paperwork completed so VA could execute the transfer.

—By mid-quarter, arrange with GRCC instructors to take finals as soon as possible (hope for an early getaway, hit the trail for Oregon sooner).

Then out of nowhere, Tina announces she isn't moving to K-Falls.

You know how, when you're kicked in the gut you can't move or breathe or speak? I just got kicked. I finally managed to exhale, "Why?"

In a voicetone that froze the air between us she spat, "What are you doing? Deliberately sabotaging *my* chances to get *my* degree?"

"I have no intention of doing that," I said calmly. "We checked out the drafting program at OIT, remember, and found that you could transfer directly into it with no loss of credit."

"You could wait here for me to finish my program at Green River first."

"Tina, I can't do that. If I'm to get my engineering degree, I have to go right now to K-Falls. If I miss even a term I lose the VA grant forever. Those are the rules." When she didn't answer I continued. "Look, Hon. You can stay on here with Mom and Dad. You finish your course and I'll start mine. We can still get together on weekends."

"That's not acceptable," she said.

Now just what the hell, I wondered, is Tina's real problem here?

I never got an answer. My wife just packed up herself and our baby and left for New York to be with her parents. She simply packed and left. In the middle of the term. Without even finishing the classes she had just claimed were so important to her.

Christ, I thought, what is happening to her? Ever since she had the baby she had gotten more and more of a pain to live with. It was like extended — permanent, maybe — post-partum depression. I had done my best to rationalize these attitudes she was coming up with, but damn, this was out of hand. This was not the lady I married four years ago.

7

In March of 1981 I finished the term at Green River Community College, received my Associate in Drafting degree, and moved to Klamath Falls. Gary, a classmate and friend from Green River, also transferred to Oregon Institute of Technology to enroll in the electronic engineering degree program. I moved into the (inexpensive!) three-bedroom apartment I had procured and signed for — except instead of living there with my wife and child I shared it with Gary.

Actually, after I was settled in I tried to get Tina to come back to the West Coast so we could be a family again, but she refused. So I decided to let her have her space for a while and maybe she would come to her senses.

Spring term at OIT was a total bomb-out. Compared to GRCC's laid-back expectations of student performance, OIT was an extreme heavyweight. I took what I thought to be a reasonable load for my first term in a new school and I got wiped out. Straight D's and F's. The Crohn's problem worsened. Nights were largely sleepless. I had flashbacks about that damned war. The ghosts made their nightly visits. God, how I wish they would leave me alone!

There was the same old thing about meeting new people and not being able to identify with them, so the making of friends hung in limbo and I felt like an oddball who couldn't assimilate into the civilian world. And the worst stress of all—or maybe what caused all the rest of it—was the absence of my loving wife and beautiful baby. God, how I missed them!

My downfall with OIT was that I didn't have an academic adviser. The person who's supposed to take care of that is the VA voc rehab counselor—and he didn't show up until halfway through the term. When he did appear he acted like it was a big imposition to make the trip all the way from Portland to the bottom of the state to meet us veterans (K-Falls is about six miles from the California border). Where Dan Southerland had been concerned about my progress and genuinely interested in how I was getting along, this new dude seemed to care about nothing except a fast wrap-up of his sessions with us vets and getting out of the area.

This jerk did nothing to help me get an academic advisor. Nor was he interested in directing me to a doctor. Since there is no VA medical facility within a hundred miles, he informed me that I could "go to any local doctor as long as the bill did not exceed $52 a month." Which meant no medical care at all, because fifty-two dollars can't begin to cover treatment for Crohn's disease, x-rays, and lab work.

What good was this guy? What good was the Oregon VA?

In the summer, Tina came back.

Andrea was happy to be back with Daddy. I was relieved and grateful that she even remembered me.

Tina was ... different. Strange and aloof. She was not the lovely, steel-anchor lady I married.

Tina, Gary, and I found a huge four-bedroom house in the small, nearby community of Midland. Three-twenty-five a month. It was out in the country, clean and clear and peaceful, and it had a fabulous view of Mt. Shasta. God, how I loved it! But for the pit-bottom economy, I could easily make my home here forever. Make no mistake, this has to be one of the most beautiful parts of this country.

Tina and I got the master bedroom, Andrea had her own room, and Gary took the bedroom near the utility room, where he had almost total privacy and he could come and go as he pleased. The fourth bedroom we turned into our study and class-project lab.

Despite all our space and all the beauty surrounding us, Tina seemed unhappy.

I ended up blowing the summer term, too.

In the student center one day I talked one day with Craig Yarborough, another Nam vet.

"Practically every Vietnam vet has the same set of common problems," Craig told me. "Losing the ability to concentrate.

Flashbacks. Jitters, jumps, sudden uncontrollable rage. In pop psych, all the symptoms are lumped together and called Post Traumatic Stress Disorder. Seems like most vets try to deny they have it because nobody wants to think he needs a shrink. Mostly what a guy needs to do is just talk about it with someone else who understands."

I sipped my coffee without answering. I was curious to see where Craig was going with this.

"There's a group of us who meet regularly for counseling," Craig went on, "and to ... well, you know, just talk about it."

The war is indeed still in you. You have not yet put it in the past. God, could you really be one of those Nam wackos you hear about in the news?

I knew I was what people called anti-social. I knew I couldn't get comfortable with situations I could not control—and I wasn't much in control of anything lately. I was scared about myself, and for my family. But I thought I did a pretty good job of covering it up.

"Do I look like I'm stressed out?" I asked, trying to sound nonchalant and casual.

"For whatever it's worth," Craig said, "we all have post-traumatic stress disorder of varying degrees and frequency. Seems strange the VA recognizes the problem enough to give it a name but not a rating. There's no disability rating for PTSD, you know. But the VA will pay for the counseling services."

Craig paused. "Some of us guys meet in a PTSD counseling group. Want to come with me?"

After giving it some thought I decided what the heck; it couldn't hurt. So I gave it a try.

The shrink, as it turned out, was actually a minister. After all, this guy never served in the military let alone experienced combat. But I gave him his chance.

We hit it off from the get-go. By his personality, his sincere interest, and his probing but nonconfrontational questioning, he got me to start to open up about my experiences in Nam. Most important, he didn't pass judgment.

He got me to think. Focus.

"Do you sleep well?" *No.*

"Do you have flashbacks to Vietnam?" *Yes, and getting worse.*

"Difficulty concentrating?" *Yes, especially lately.*

"Drug or alcohol abuse?" *I'm grateful to be one of the few vets that doesn't have a D&A problem. I'm not lily-white; I've been known to get tanked, but I never looked for an answer in a bottle. Been known to buy a six-pack and have some left a month later. Never did any dope. None. Ever. Just don't mess with my cigarettes and coffee!*

"Difficulty developing relationships with people?" *I get pissed off when people get bent about trivial things, the games people play, a whole society that creates people afraid to be themselves. I can't stand phonies, the lack of personal values, the absence of principles and commitment. I just get damn weary of all the bullshit people sling.*

"Guilt about surviving when others did not?" *Of course. How and why did I survive? I witnessed so much death and destruction, had so many narrow escapes. At one point I wanted to die over there.*

"Unexpected anger? Violence?" *I am aware, and I take care. I've trashed out my share of furniture and dishes. If I got into a scuffle, the scuffler would fight to kick my ass and I would fight to kill. That really scares me. I avoid putting myself in those positions. I don't go to bars or other places where someone under the influence might start something.*

"Suspicious or afraid of people? Do you avoid crowds?" *Many times while driving down a stretch of highway I'm looking for possible ambush locations. In a restaurant, I must be seated in a booth with my back to the wall. I can not make myself wait in a long line; I have walked out of a grocery store leaving a full cart in the aisle rather than wait in a long checkout line.*

"Do you think Vietnam has affected your life?" *Oh, God, I had not realized how much. Vietnam is what I am. It is still deeply imbedded in me. The training and the mentality developed for survival back then is still with me.*

After a month of private sessions, the counselor took me to his group meetings. Suddenly I found I was not alone. I was not a fruitcake, after all. Vietnam, and the way we were treated afterward, affected the lives of everyone who served there. And that was why we were all in therapy. I began to open up and get things off my chest that had been nagging me for years.

Every other session was husbands and wives (or "significant others") together, and Tina went to those sessions with me. It was important that spouses learn to understand PTSD, to understand it was a common denominator for us all, how it effected marriages and families, and how to cope with all of it. The wives said it was really helpful to them. Tina went to those sessions with me.

There was one big problem about Tina. She lied through her teeth about me.

"What does Chuck do that really upsets you?" the therapist asked.

Tina responded with totally fabricated stories. Chuck has a terrible temper. He hits, curses, throws things. Chuck snaps at our little girl for nothing; he's a tightwad; he's scornful and rude to my parents, a poor provider, won't meet his family responsibilities, doesn't allow me my freedom.

I had no response. I couldn't tell the group she was lying; I would be accused of avoiding the issue, of not facing reality.

These changes in Tina — her awful moodiness, her antagonism toward me: What if she were not salvageable as a person? As I tried hard to analyze it, I realized the changes seemed to revolve around the birth of Andrea.

"Stop crying! Stop whining. Eat. Get to bed. Shut up!" she screamed at Andrea, time and again. "I hate you! I wish you were never born!"

I tried to intervene. "Don't you dare talk to my daughter like that. You don't treat *any* child like that."

Each time, Tina turned on me. "Stay out of it, stupid freaking sonofabitchin' asshole." Or, "Get out and stop interfering I'm in charge here don't you dare put me down in front of my daughter."

While I was in the Army, before little Andrea came into our lives, our relationship was a thing of beauty, the envy of many. We were carefree and happy, even with the few material things we had. Andrea brought a new level of responsibility, someone other than our selves to revolve around. And belt-tightening. I went for over a year without buying myself so much as a pair of shoes. That was okay; I was happy to sacrifice my needs to my wife and daughter. It made me a provider; it made me fatherly.

Tina, on the other hand, was unable to adjust to selflessness, that she considered Andrea an inconvenience. Tina put on the good show when anyone else was around—in retrospect, I see this as the beginning of her life as an actress; but alone within our own home she was unmercifully rough on the poor child.

I still had no appointment for a hearing before the Board of Veterans Appeals. I sent an inquiry and received this cutesy little note of evasion:

Your application for benefits has been received and you will be notified when further action is necessary.

So. The VA is telling me they are doing nothing. I am still in hang fire mode.

The United States Government sent the United States Marines to Lebanon. The United States Government called it a Peace Keeping Force.

In the Student Center at Oregon Institute of Technology I sipped coffee while I waited for Tina to get out of class. A couple of ROTC students joined me, wanting to talk about the presence of the Marines in Lebanon, and my thoughts about it.

"They are going to die!" My automatic response erupted without forethought, and I shocked myself with my own abruptness.

The surprised future military leaders assailed me with questions. "How do you know? Why do you think so?"

"It's just like Vietnam," I explained. "First of all, our military is getting into something without understanding the culture. Muslims really believe in suicide in the name of Allah. It is common for them to launch suicide attacks. And knowing our military as I do, I doubt our guards have live ammunition, and if they do, it isn't loaded in their weapons.

"Secondly," I continued, "as I saw it on the news, all the American troops are being housed in a single building. That breaks one of the first tactical rules of combat or any hostile environment: Never allow your people to be clustered in one large group or in one location."

"So?" a cadet prompted. "That means they die?"

"Figure it out," I said. "Either a suicide plane loaded with explosives will destroy the building by crashing into it, or several of them swoop down and hammer it. Of course there is the chance of a massive artillery barrage, or even a car bomb."

"Our military leaders wouldn't let that happen," protested the future military leaders drinking coffee in the college Student Center.

"It already did happen," I said. *Christ, don't these kids pay attention to the news?* "Other targets in that region, including our Embassy, have already been attacked. Our military leaders may be very intelligent in other things, but they tend not to pay attention to history. We are constantly being kicked in the butt by doing things history has proven we shouldn't. We know the enemies' capabilities and still disregard them, because we are the Almighty American Military and you can't show us anything we don't already know."

"No way, Lewis!" protested the Kid Cadets. "Our brass knows what it's doing!"

"Yes, just like the brass knew what it was doing in Nam." *Jesus H. Christ, don't they teach these warriors about war?* "You see, it is now historical fact that part of our undoing in Vietnam was our lack of information about the Vietnamese culture and mentality. If we had a better understanding of that, we would have had a better understanding of what we up against. We would not have been stumbling through the jungle looking for what we thought was the enemy.

"And as for our service men in Lebanon," I went on, circling around to the point at hand, "the American serviceman is spoiled. He has to have his luxuries, like a nice building with all the amenities. This is the wrong concept for men in a combat zone. Like it or not, right now Lebanon is a combat zone."

Later that same week came the tragic news that the Marine barracks was destroyed by a suicide driver with a car bomb.

The news affected me deeply. I wanted to scream at the world; I wanted to cry with the ones who lost sons and husbands so needlessly. I prayed for the immediate court martial of the commanders in charge. The stupid bastards should have foreseen it; this was nothing short of gross negligence and incompetence on their part. Once again the shining pride of America's youth had to pay the ultimate price because their leaders were more interested in politics and career advancement than in being military leaders. God damn them, damn them all!

When the first news reports came in, the ROTC boys sought me out to apologize.

Rather than hemming and hawing with false humility, I took the opportunity to drive home a point. "It is a sorry state when an ex-NCO who has been out of the Army for almost four years can identify a threat that active generals either don't see or won't take seriously," I told them, and I couldn't resist adding, "Generals Patton and Bradley and our other exemplary past military leaders must be rolling over in their graves."

I looked the young cadets square in the eye and told them, "Take this awful event as an example, but do not take it as exemplary. Today's military brass is so wrapped in their own career management and advancement that they forget they are, first and foremost, LEADERS, and responsible for the lives of the men in their command. This sheer folly is a senseless waste of America's youth."

The horrors of Vietnam returned, full focus. I was again haunted by the needless sacrifice my brothers at arms were forced to make because of politically based military leadership. When will generals and politicians quit trying to do each others' jobs? Until they do, we will continue to kill and maim our youth as they are sent where they should not go, to interfere in the battles of other peoples they do not understand.

In August I began scraping, saving, and stashing nickels and dimes in an effort to show my wife how much I loved her. I began planning a special anniversary celebration for her, and I had until December 23 to pull it off.

I bought the diamond ring Tina had never had. A friend's wife helped me select a dazzling evening dress and all the trappings. I hired a sitter, made a reservation at the best-slash-most expensive restaurant in town, booked the honeymoon suite at the local Best Western and had the room appointed with roses, carnations, champagne, and good wine.

I had a lot of help from friends, most of whom were in my PTSD counseling group, and who, therefore, understood the domestic stress and related to it and to me. They recommended places, suggested stores, referred a baby sitter, and "absentmindedly" left change on the table when they joined me at the Student Center.

On December 23 I went about my day as usual ... until it was time to start celebrating. I presented Tina with her new gown and told her a bigger surprise was yet to come.

"What's this?!" she demanded.

I asked her to just put it on and get ready for a special evening. She walked away grumbling something.

At the restaurant everything was perfect, from the selection of our table to the waitress bringing the diamond ring and card along with our wine before dinner.

Tina took the card and opened it, her sour expression never leaving her face. Then she opened the little box.

Tina looked at the ring in its presentation box, then she looked at me with ... disdain, and her voice was ... flat and cold. "This is all a stupid waste."

Not another word was spoken through the rest of the meal. But then, how can a man speak when he has been blown out of the water and kicked in the teeth and balls?

At the door of the restaurant, Tina commanded, "Take me to the movie."

A diamond ring, and she wants to go see a B-grade?

After the movie I took her to the honeymoon suite. She ignored it all. No comment, no thank you. Without so much as glancing around, dropped into bed and fell asleep. Hell, I should have taken her home and slept in the motel by myself.

Nothing she could do could have hurt me more.

Naturally, all my friends who helped plan the event asked how it went. I wanted to lie, to tell them it was beautiful, but I couldn't. I told it as it happened.

Craig's wife, the woman who helped select Tina's dress, placed a hand on my arm. "Now we see what you have endured, Chuck, and now we all know now about Tina's lies. We see what she is."

"I love her," I insisted. "I just need more counseling so I'll know how to reach her."

"She's the one needing counseling, Chuck," Craig said.

Finally, I gathered enough nerve to speak to Tina. "Why did you act like that on our anniversary?"

Each of her words was an ice pick stabbing my heart. "You can never buy my emotions that easily."

BUY her emotions? My God, this woman has no idea that I am in love with her.

During the next session of group counseling everyone asked Tina what she thought of my anniversary surprise, though through the gossip line they already knew what happened. Some of them had seen how she acted in the restaurant, including Gary, who worked there part time. Tina, not realizing they played a big role in helping me, told them it was "great" and "fantastic." Now Tina was caught in her lie. Now everyone in the group had her number.

I had no sense of accomplishment over Tina's personal pain at being exposed. But if nothing else, it showed her as the liar she was. Now everyone knew for sure that I was not as bad as she was trying to make me look. And yes, there was satisfaction in that.

8

"Your academic record at OIT is lousy, Mr. Lewis, and your progress ... there isn't any."

It was the beginning of winter term when my itinerant VA voc rehab counselor made one of his rare appearances on campus. Now I was on his carpet.

"You still have not connected me with an academic adviser, and I am the first to admit I have floundered on my own wings. I need guidance, and I'm not getting any, neither from VA Vocational Rehabilitation *(that means you, you lazy S.O.B.)* nor from the school *(which you were supposed to arrange)*. I guess the voc rehab counselor in Washington state spoiled me with his total supportiveness *(which is my polite way of saying you haven't done squat for the vets here, you imbecile)*. Then, too, Voc Rehab hasn't arranged for a doctor to treat—"

"I intend to close your case and withdraw you from the program," he interrupted. Then, taking on a fake-conciliatory tone, he added, "First, however, you must be interviewed by a psychologist before we can drop you from the program."

So! YOU don't have all this one-man power, after all. Egotist.

"I will set up your appointment, and you must keep it without excuse and without fail."

"All right, I'll see the shrink. But I am sure I will prove myself this term."

"At this point that's immaterial." *He means he doesn't care.* "I am dropping you from school effective the end of this term. If, however, you do happen to get it together this term, which I doubt, I might consider reinstating you, which is doubtful also."

Damn, this guy had no interest in me from the start. I wonder how many other vets' lives he's screwing with.

My appointment was right in the middle of mid-terms. At OIT, the only acceptable excuse for missing mid-term or final exams was ... none at all. Was this Mr. God-playing VA Counselor's way of making *sure* I scrubbed another term? As it happened, I was pretty close to flub-proof this quarter. Straight B's, every class. Okay, I thought, I will just arrange to take my mid-terms early.

The shrink was at the VA facility in White City, Oregon, a hundred and fifty mile drive from K-Falls. First, road construction delays. Then, I got lost—in that tiny little berg! As a result I was a half-hour late for the appointment, and as a result of *that,* I was in a bad mood the minute I walked in.

Being late didn't mean much; I still had to wait almost an hour.

After almost five hours of tests and interviews, I was told to go outside and wait. I waited by napping in the car. Then came the summons to reappear for discussion of the results of the tests.

The shrink delivered a long spiel in psychobabble, which in plain English meant I do in fact have Post Traumatic Stress Disorder. "I strongly recommend you undergoing counseling immediately," he added.

"I am in counseling, have been for almost six months," I replied, then explained the program at K-Falls.

He stroked his chin, classic shrinker-thinker fashion. "Mmm. You really require sophisticated, more fully professional help than that program is apparently designed to deliver. But for the immediate duration, your present regimen provides at least a measure of the connectivity so essential to you at this time."

I defended my friends and my counselor. "I am more connected to those people than I have ever been to anyone."

"Good; that's good. Mr. Lewis, according to the fairly extensive and quite reliable profile we have derived from your various tests today, your training and experience make you one of the most latently dangerous people I know, in my judgment. You have the fullest capability to spontaneously carry out a rampage that could end in massive destruction. You would be cognizant and in control through the very end, until you end up dead yourself."

Ouch! I started to bristle inside but I quickly corked it. This guy had just pretty much slashed me up but I didn't feel like giving him the satisfaction of getting to see me erupt. So I calmly asked, "I'm a walking time bomb?"

"When and if you should explode, I would just as soon be in another state."

I remained calm. "Well, sir, the United States Military trains us to kill, then presents with honors and awards for doing it. It's our job, for Christ sake. But I hardly feel I am a threat to anyone outside the confines of war."

"On the positive side, Mr. Lewis, you are a shoo-in candidate for a disability award for Post Traumatic Stress Disorder."

"Shit. From whom? The VA? The government recognizes the problem but they don't award *anything* for PTSD. Hundreds of veterans have applied for PTSD compensation, and not a damned one has received anything."

Besides, the morons at VA can't even understand I have Crohn's, and *that* can be proven with testing. How could anyone expect a disability rating for something *not* physical?
I kept my thoughts to myself, though, lest I give this guy the idea that I'm paranoid—in addition to being dangerous.

Then from the mouth of God, Junior came the *coup de Gras.* "It is my belief, Mr. Lewis, that you are incapable of completing school at Oregon Institute of Technology. Frankly, I am amazed that you graduated Green River at all, let alone doing so with honors."

Now you are not capable of being educated, Lewis. You don't have the ability to learn academics.

I knew now that this guy was full of shit.

I knew, too, that my schooling was kicked in the ass, as soon as the shrink's narrative got to my VA adviser.

On the way home the trash tossed itself off the walls of my mind. I'm trying to go to school, care for a family, going to counseling to throw off the ghosts of war, fighting an incurable disease, fighting the VA for my rightful entitlements, losing the woman I love. Of course I'm dealing with stress, dammit! But my problems are nowhere near what this clown was trying to lay on me. Screw him, and the camel he rode in on.

Okay, Lewis. Stop wallowing in it. Options, please.

Work. It's overdue time I got back to work anyway.

Crohn's Disease equals unemployability. You found that out already.

Hell with that excuse. I didn't try hard enough, or I looked in the wrong places. Maybe I didn't dress right for interviews; maybe I used the wrong mouth wash.

Where is the right place? The Pacific Northwest is wrapped up in Boeing Aircraft ... Boeing, farming, and timber. Lord, if I can't handle a calf or a pony, I sure couldn't wrestle a plane or a fir tree.

Back east. I've heard jobs are plentiful there. The New York vicinity—Tina would be closer to her family, maybe bring her out of whatever is troubling her.

Then lay it out like it's all for her. But no matter how you tell it, she'll accuse you of trying to sabotage her schooling—again. And you can't afford to hang around K-Falls while she finishes; there's no work there.

Hey, listen, there are community colleges on every fourth corner in Jersey, Pennsylvania, New York. Surely one of them has a great drafting program. She'll love the prestige of attending an "East Coast School."

Okay, then figure out how you're going to confront Tina with this latest blow to our lives.

That is going to be very difficult, because ever since our anniversary my wife has not even discussed our grocery list in a civil manner.

Tina had just put Andrea in bed, but true to her routine my girl wasn't going to sleep without seeing her daddy. I told her a very condensed story, gave her a hug and two kisses and closed her door. Then I went out to tell my wife her life was about to change again.

I sat Tina in front of the fireplace, then gave her the blow-by-blow account of my day at the shrink parlor. To my astonishment, she listened all the way through, silently and without her usual butting-in.

"New York! Chuck, that's terrific! You go to work and I'll go to school! We'll make it all so wonderful!"

I was shocked speechless.

"But that shrink," she went on, butting in on my speechlessness. "He isn't worth the powder to blow his nose. Sure, you have some problems. All Nam vets have problems. Yours are nowhere near the magnitude the shrink or that VA guy are trying to make them."

So why did you tell the counseling group they are?

Even with Tina's acceptance and enthusiasm, I was down, way down. Never before had I failed, never before quit. I had let my family down, because instead of becoming an engineer, I would be a median-wage draftsman.

In three weeks we had severed our ties in Klamath Falls and coordinated our immediate arrangements with Tina's family in New York. I bolstered my spirits with visions of escorting Tina to Broadway shows, to museums and places of the fine arts, of showing my uptown wife that I, too, had class and style. If anyone wants to do the style thing, New York City is the place to do it.

I traded the Mustang for a long-bed van. We set the van up to be our mobile residence en route — food, drinks, Andrea's toys, and creature-comfort items. The rest of our belongings went to storage, with arrangements for the movers to send them along when we got settled in the Big Apple.

In the middle of March of 1983, Tina and I and an almost-two-years-old Andrea arrived in New York City, but not with the hoorah I expected. An unexpected, inexplicable iciness hung between Tina and her parents.

9

The second day in New York I landed a job interview.

Alex, the owner of the company, kept me on the phone for over an hour. I had all the answers to his questions. When I hung up, I felt sure the phone conversation nailed the job, and that the interview, set for the following day, was just a formality.

I decided to bring Tina with me to the interview, because I was lost in the city. I went to get the van, warm it up, and bring it around to the front of my in-laws' apartment building. Tina took an unexpectedly long time to get to the van. When she did slip into the passenger seat she was crying.

"Pop's not happy we're here," she finally sobbed after a lot of coaxing. "He called my husband a lowlife. I said you are not, that you're really trying, you're a disabled American veteran, that you got a job interview right away and we aren't here to sponge."

Yeah, disabled while defending the old codger's right to despise me.

Both of us were angry and perplexed, but we focused on the job at hand. We arrived at the site I hoped would be my new place of work.

It turned out to be a factory and it was my first taste of New York City's fear of itself. Security was so tight and entrances to the building so camouflaged I couldn't figure out how to get in. As I stood outside pondering my situation, the door to the loading dock opened. I hailed the employee at the door, told him who I was and that I had an appointment with Alex. The gentleman took me in and introduced me to Steve, who, among a whole list of titles and duties, was Alex's shop manager.

Alex manufactured lighting fixtures. A look around and my mind spun with the creative opportunities here and my interest was captured in moments.

And I was right: I was hired. On the spot. I was to begin Monday morning.

That evening Tina and I took turns finishing each others' sentences in telling Pop about my job, and, gloating silently, I watched him eat the crow. What made it more fun was that he didn't know I knew he was having to eat it.

I prepared for my new job by getting a new battery for the van, driving practice runs from Pop's place to Alex's, and buying some decent clothes to attire myself properly for working in an office. My wardrobe of beat-up jeans and ratty workshirts didn't fit my new-found station.

Alex was one hell of a guy to work for. He and Steve let me do my job without hovering and with no interference. He explained. He taught. Ditto Steve. They made me so comfortable I never hesitated to ask questions. "No, your questions are not stupid," Steve once told me. "You have to know something before you can frame the proper question."

I had been there only two months when Alex sent me to the Illuminating Engineering Society's lighting education program—at company expense. I quickly learned that there is a hell of a lot more to lighting than simply flipping a switch. Alex originally hired me as a draftsman, but it wasn't long before I was in charge of a production line as well as doing research and development with some new lamps on the market. I also worked as a purchaser, and assisted in putting the factory on line with a computer-controlled system. All this excitement, learning, and involvement, plus, given my lack of experience, a very fair pay and benefits package.

Steve and I ran the factory in general, while Alex brought in the business, did the client contact work, and was administrator. There was a good karma between Alex, Steve and me, so that before long we covered and complemented. If one was out the other could get the job done. As CEO, Alex may have had his worries, but plant operations was not one of them.

I only hoped I had time to establish myself before the next debilitating Crohn's flare-up.

Perhaps it was being near her mom and pop (despite his stated dislike of me), but Tina mellowed out. She began to resemble the woman I fell in love with. Now our biggest problem was finding a place to live. In New York City housing is ridiculous.

I have never seen such filth or shoddy housing. The five-to-six-hundred-dollar range, in Seattle, would get us a palace; in New York City, it wouldn't get a place fit for my dog.

People in the lower income brackets—working people—don't stand a chance in the Big Apple. Greedy landlords charge absolutely criminal prices and fees for rent and related expenses. A townhouse apartment almost identical to the one we rented in Auburn, Washington for $375 a month went for $1800 in NYC. What working person can afford that? Who can afford to get out of the projects and reestablish elsewhere?

We struck a rent and board and household expense agreement with Tina's parents. At least her pop could not claim we were mooching, sponging, and freeloading. Pay him generously though I did, nothing I could do seemed to impress him. But what the hell, I figured, in due time I would prove I was better than the old buzzard thought I was.

Alex showed his extraordinariness as both an employer and a human being when he not only listened with empathy and understanding to my plight with the VA, but when, after only two weeks in his employ, he gave me a day off to transfer my records from Oregon to New York.

I did not, however, give him the complete details of the Crohn's Disease. I was having problems but managed to hide it. I should have leveled with him from the start, but I was getting by and he didn't mention my constant trips to the men's room.

The NYC VA office initiated the process of transferring my records to the city. Everything else, they told me, could be done by phone, eliminating the need to miss work. Service connected medical problems would be treated at Kingbridge Medical Center in Bronx.

After little more than two months at work my back popped. When I tried to work anyway, Alex told me to get to a doctor.

"You're a month away from being on the company insurance plan, Chuck, but I'm willing to stretch your date of employment," Alex said.

"No," I declined. "My back injury is service connected. It would be useful to have information about recurring problems on my record. I'll go to the VA facility at Kingbridge."

Kingbridge personnel were very courteous, a far cry from the hostility shown in Seattle. Kingbridge doctors put me through all sorts of tests and evaluations. They had equipment the Army didn't, but they still couldn't nail down the source of my pain.

I was also having an exacerbation of the Crohn's. If I had to have a flare-up, this was the opportune time for one. So I requested an examination.

"Crohn's Disease, if you have it, which here looks like it's doubtful, is listed as non-service connected," said the doc, scanning my record. "We can neither examine nor treat you at this time."

Despite what my records said, I continued to press the Crohn's issue every time I saw a doctor. I thought if I complained about it enough—it's been five years now—someone would finally give it a serious look.

I called the regional VA office. "Our hands are tied until your appeal has been processed," said the chipper, phone-side voice.

"Could you please check on the status of my appeal?"

"I'm afraid that information is not available at this time."

"I would appreciate it if you would please look into it, let me know if there is any sort of problem I should know about," I said. What I actually meant was *You people don't really care!*

I am starting to develop a serious attitude problem with the VA in general. I appreciate what they are doing for my back, but I also need attention for the Crohn's. I need to find a diversion to prevent me from dwelling too much on all this outrageous indifference and incompetence .

10

After coming home from the Vietnam War most vets sought security, solace, and comradeship in the various veterans service organizations. However, most of the large mainstream organizations did not accept us; or they were willing to accept our membership fees but made it clear our participation was not wanted. Those groups simply did not consider Vietnam was a real war nor Nam vets to be real veterans. The older WW II and Korean War types wanted nothing to do with this new generation of youthful warriors. We Nam vets had no place to turn, no organization to belong to. Such organizations were needed desperately, and probably could have helped many a Nam vet through the transition of being back in the world again, and to help him deal with PTSD.

Finally a group of Nam vets formed an organization of their own. Hence the Vietnam Veterans of America Inc. (VVA) was formed and obtained its Congressional charter.

The Vietnam Veterans of America had a chapter nearby and, intending to join the organization, I went to a meeting. The guest speaker was one of the attorneys representing Vietnam vets in the Agent Orange lawsuit against the government.

As he attempted to explain the suit's progress the VVA membership ripped him apart, taking exception to each point and barraging him with hostile questions and antagonistic remarks. I heard not one voice in support of this man who, with his associates, on his own time and with his own money, was fighting the Nam vets' war for them. After being treated with unspeakable rudeness, the invited guest did not even get a thank-you.

That evening I was ashamed to call myself a Vietnam veteran. If it were I, I would have told the ungrateful asses to go fight their own suit and pay for it themselves.

Battling the consequences of Agent Orange myself, I support the lawsuit fully. Our government must be held responsible for exposing its citizens to those hazards, and so must the chemical companies involved. Those firms sold untried toxins to the government without knowing what its side effects may be, and the government sprayed it all over Vietnam without knowing, either. Oh, yes, the government and the companies were negligent, without a doubt. The chem firms wanted to make some serious money, and the government bought unknown shit in the name of bringing the war to an end sooner and saving American lives by denying the enemy vegetation to hide in.

After the meeting I introduced myself to the attorney. "I for one appreciate what you are doing," I told him. "Given the circumstances I think you and your associates are doing the best that can be expected. Unfortunately, what we vets can expect is ... to lose. You don't just up and haul the U.S. Government and the most powerful chemical companies in this land into court and actually expect to flat-out win. Not with their unlimited financial resources and all the stall tactics the system allows them."

The legal-eagle looked a little puzzled that anyone would give him any kudos after such a hostile reaction. So I tried to explain myself. "I'm sorry for the reception you got here, and I am appalled and embarrassed. What I witnessed was selfish and self destructive. I am no member here but I came intending to join this brotherhood. But these ungrateful morons are no brothers of mine." As we shook hands in departure, I added, "I need to be active in a productive cause and organization, but this is obviously not it."

I couldn't have been more satisfied with my job or all the people I worked with. I did my damnedest to keep the Crohn's hidden from the boss but I couldn't hide my back ailment. When the Crohn's had me doubled up with cramping I said it was from the back. I shouldn't have lied to Alex; in hindsight I know he would have accepted what was.

Meanwhile, Tina found a job on a production line. Hard work, piss pay. Her earnings should have helped our family's finances but as things ended up, she spent all her income on her own special projects. Clothes for herself, frills for Andrea, going and doing with her mom and pop—proving herself the big-city cultured personality, which turned out to cost all her income plus a big and unaffordable bite of mine. I found myself forced into doing things in the name of "family;" if I didn't participate Tina and the old folks belittled me as anti-social.

Pop expected house and family to revolve around his diabetes. "You have to show consideration of my condition," he insisted. My own "condition," though, he dismissed as fabrications.

What you should do, Chuck, is go along on one of the old bastard's outings when you're flaring up. Then shit all over yourself in the car.

They all made it clear I was to go with them for a lakeside picnic on the Fourth of July. The old folks, ourselves, and Tina's two sisters and their men and children. It was going to be a nightmare: I knew that despite fireworks being illegal in New York state, there would be fireworks. Like so many vets, I still have that startle reflex from pops, bangs, loud noises, and explosions.

We got to the Upstate lake by seven in the morning, and already the parking lot was packed with (it seemed like) all of New York City. Fireworks exploded all around, and park security wasn't doing a damn thing about it. I was a nervous wreck by eight o'clock and by noon I was emotionally back in the field of battle.

From the top of the hillside, some kids started throwing fireworks directly at us. I cracked. I went after the little shits. Luckily for them they got away. Soon I spotted another gang of little snots, saw them light the fuse and aim. I grabbed my six-month-old nephew and whirled around, putting myself between him and the firecracker. It hit and exploded where his head had rested, burning a hole in his blanket. No mere ladyfinger, this; it was serious fireworks.

Then I exploded. I roared straight up the hillside, forget the winding trail leading to the top, pursuing those little brats as they fled.

"Grandpa, Grandpa! This mean man is going to beat us up!" they wailed.

These kids are ... what? Eight? Nine? Is this the guy who let them play with firecrackers?

I grabbed Grandpa by the throat and told him what had just happened. "And if you don't do something about it, I will," I promised.

Grandma croaked something about "killing my husband" and dashed off to "get the cops."

"Fine. Go ahead," I said, giving Grandpa another neck shake. "I haven't committed a crime. Yet. But you have. Fireworks are illegal. Not supervising children is illegal. Attempting to murder a baby is, too, last time I looked."

"Yes, yes, I'll deal with my boys!" Grandpa said pleadingly, fumbling with his glasses I had shaken askew. "It won't ever happen again, I swear it."

My nephew's father, arriving on the run, pulled me off the irresponsible old fart. I kept on yelling about kids being too young to handle major fireworks, about adults setting rotten examples about flaunting the law. I was having a stone fit, and I think if not for Tom's intervention I would have hurt that old fart.

In the meantime Tina found a cop ... and *she* filed a formal complaint ... about *me!* She said the guilty kids needed protection from *me*.

Tom and I and Tina and the cop converged at our picnic spot at the same time. I explained what happened and showed the officer where the firecracker burned the blanket. I told him about the confrontation with the hoodlums' grandfather.

"Well, you know how boys will be boys," the cop intoned behind his protective wall of sunglasses and pasted-on grin. "Got to control the temper there, sir, don't spoil the spirit of the Fourth." He unlocked my gaze and nodded at everyone in general. "You folks have a nice day, he ordered." Then the guardian of justice strolled off to protect some more citizens.

"Chuck, you stupid idiot, what the hell you tryin' to do?" my father-in-law exploded. "Chasin' innocent little kids, jumpin' all over people, threatenin' t' kill 'em?"

"Jesus God Almighty, Pop! First of all I didn't threaten to kill anyone. Kick some well deserved ass, maybe, but not kill. Second, those 'innocent little kids' could have killed your grandson. And that's a minor little no big deal?" *How did things suddenly turn unreal?* "Tell you what, Pop. Next time a firecracker lands on your grandchild I do nothing. I let it explode."

"Aw, c'mon now. No use stirring up waves when you can stay quiet and keep the waters calm."

God, I have to get away from this. I left the family and spent the rest of the day in the woods, away from everything.

Why am I the bad guy here? Flashbacks. You're in the battlefield and you're responsible for the safety of your own.

I go out of my way to avoid trouble. But never back down if it comes looking for you. That's the way of a soldier.

That's the way of a New Yorker, too. You take care of yourself because nobody else, including the authorities paid to, will. You run into clowns like those kids and their grandparents. Do whatever suits their fancy and to hell with everyone else, and the system does nothing about it.

1983 turned into 1984, spring sprouted, and Tina handed me a hell of a surprise.

I was about to become a father again.

I hop-stepped all around Cloud Nine. Now Andrea would have the sibling she wanted, and I dared hope for a son to do things with.

I was also nervous. Recently, there were news leaks that Agent Orange was responsible for birth defects.

A couple of months into her pregnancy, Tina began bleeding. And bleeding. She weakened. Six, seven times, maybe more, I rushed her to the emergency room.

"She's probably just threatening to miscarry," her doctor told me when I asked the worried questions.

"*Just* miscarrying?"

"Everything is going to be all right, Mr. Lewis, I assure you. We'll keep your wife in bedrest, good nutrition, minimum activity."

We will?

"We" did what the doctor said and then Tina got *really* bad. Unable to stand my wife's being in such pain, I called the doctor from work.

"Absolutely nothing to worry about," said the doc. "Mrs. Lewis's pregnancy is perfectly normal."

I told Alex what the doctor said. Totally frustrated, I railed, "*Normal?* Normal for what? Even animals aren't allowed to suffer like this! At the present rate, my wife is going to *die* from a 'normal' pregnancy, Alex!"

Himself a father, Alex soothed, "Take the rest of the day off and get your wife to another doctor. It's obvious that something's wrong and she needs help, *now*."

I called a different doctor at another clinic, explained, said I feared it was a life-and-death emergency, and was admitted immediately. The doctor examined Tina and placed her in the hospital right away. His fetal reading showed that the baby was abnormal and had zero chance of surviving to term.

Tina and I wrestled with a decision neither of us particularly believed in and one we did not take lightly. Despite the messages from well intentioned right-to-lifers, there comes a time when a decision is intensely, individually personal, and it's nobody else's damned business.

The following morning, after the abortion was over, Tina's doctor flagged me in the waiting room.

"The fetus your wife carried was dead and had been dead for at least two weeks. For reasons we haven't yet determined, her system was unable to expel it."

My legs went Jell-O and I crumpled into the nearest chair. "You mean my wife was being slowly poisoned from carrying around decaying tissue — "

The doctor nodded.

" — while that other so-called 'doctor' was calling this a *NORMAL* pregnancy?"

The doctor stopped nodding and took on a pokerfaced expression, because he heard the word between the words: malpractice.

I left the hospital and went to the office of her other "doctor" to have her ass. Lucky for her, she had the day off.

Tina was allowed to go home that afternoon. As soon as we got there I called Alex and filled him in.

At work the next morning Alex called me into his office and asked me to explain everything to him once again.

"Just making sure I have the facts straight," he said after I retold the story, "because I already spoke to my personal lawyer about suing the hell out of Tina's doctor and the hospital she does her malpracticing in."

I was flabbergasted. And touched.

"In a day or two my attorney will have the facts gathered, then he'll let us know whether or not we have a case," Alex said.

In only thirty hours the attorney had his answer. "We have a great case against both doctor and hospital," the lawyer reported. "But there's a catch. It's a city hospital and the city passed a convenient little statute protecting the hospital and all its doctors from litigation. In other words," said the attorney, emphasizing each word for clarity, "the city made it illegal to file suit against its hospital."

"This is preposterous!" I exclaimed. "Is it possible to do such a thing?"

"I think it came out of New York City's bankruptcy a few years ago," Alex said. "To protect the city from further financial losses."

"Well, why stop with legalizing malpractice?" I scoffed. "Why not place the police, social services, schools, street cleaners, and everyone else under the same protective umbrella?"

Alex nodded and grinned. "Yep, the city fathers missed a big chance to completely protect *everyone* from *any* responsibility."

"The VA ... N'Yawk City ... write a law and *snap!* ... incompetence by legislation." I exhaled a forced a ha-ha. "Alex, why do I feel a new layer of cynicism coming on?"

My boss snorted. "Hell, Chuck, they *want* your cynicism. They must want it; they work real hard to earn it."

It wasn't just the city hospital and its doctors. I began thinking all the fruit in the Big Apple barrel were rotten.

Tina's parents, with their three-bolt doors always locked, afraid to go out on the street, living like prisoners in their home — they were only everyone else's reflection. And I began to be the same as they were: I felt exposed to risk everywhere except inside the apartment or workplace. I lived enough of that in Nam and I didn't need to live like that at home. Fear is a bad walking-partner.

And Andrea, now in her most formative years — bringing a child up in this environment was absolutely unacceptable and I would not do it.

Now if only I could persuade Tina that we needed to get away from this ghetto lifestyle ... No, we did not live at a ghetto address; but this fear, this feeling of ever imminent danger, this self-imposed prison — this is a ghetto lifestyle.

The discussion was easier than I anticipated because Tina quit her job. One day she decided it was boring, or an imposition on her carefree life, or whatever the hell her malcontent excuse was, and the next day she up and left. Suddenly I realized the pattern had always been there, that Tina starts something and then quits. Now, reluctantly, I admitted it. But not to her. This was not the battle to pick, or at least not the right time to pick it.

While I was stricken with the realization of this unhappy aspect of my wife's character, I also figured I may as well take advantage of it, for she was obviously ready for a change.

First I initiated a discussion about New York paranoia, leading Tina to agree, "We definitely do not want to raise our daughter in this environment."

"Then let's go back to the Northwest, where we can live without constantly looking over our shoulders and being suspicious of everyone around us," I prompted.

"It *would* be nice to live our own lives ... without ... " Tina stumbled for words. "Well, I guess I am ... getting ... kind of fed up with ... Pop's archaic rules and his ... strange concept of life."

Then, having said that much, she plunged on. "We are having a clash of cultures and lifestyles, aren't we, Chuck — them and us? Pop hasn't made any effort to understand us or our financial hard times or your situation with your health and with all the crap and inaction from the VA."

Surprised? I hoped my jaw didn't dent the carpet when it dropped to the floor. Until this moment I had no idea Tina knew of my inner conflict with her dad. Then she surprised me anew.

"To tell the truth, Chuck, I prefer living out West. New York is not the beautiful city I remember ... and ... I'm ... well, I'm ready to get out from under Pop's thumb. Ready to go back to the West Coast."

I contacted some Washington state lighting firms I had done business with on behalf of Alex's company, and within days I had two job offers.

I approached Alex with stomach knots that had nothing to do with Crohn's. Here I am, having to go to this man I like and respect, the person who gave me my life back, whose company I love working for and do not want to leave, and tell him I can't deal with anything outside the job and I'm moving. Christ, that sounds just like I'm running away. I feel guilty as hell leaving Alex; I feel like I betrayed his trust and confidence.

And all that is what I told Alex, plain and unpolished.

With grace and understanding, Alex accepted my resignation. As his final fine and thoughtful gesture, he wrote an awesome letter of recommendation. Steve did the same.

Just before departing the Big Apple I reported to the VA office, informing them of my move and requesting them to transfer my records to the Seattle regional office.

In the year's time since my initial contact with them, the New York VA communicated with me only once: to summon me for the annual quick glance they call a physical exam. An evaluation for Crohn's was not part of it. My attempt to get it recognized (and compensated) was going nowhere, and nobody cared, not the VA and not Tina's family. So why shouldn't my in-laws believe the Crohn's wasn't real, that it was nothing more than an excuse I used to avoid the city-life social happenings they were constantly setting up? If the VA wouldn't say it was so, why should Pop believe it was?

More an intent to make her remember me than a hope of getting any actual information, I asked, "Can you tell me the status of the appeal I filed last year?"

She shrugged. "Don't know."

"You could look it up."

"Don't have that information here at my desk."

"I'll wait while you get up and get it."

She got up and I waited. And waited. She was back in about the length of time it takes to drink a cup of coffee and ... well, I noticed she had reapplied her lipstick.

"Charles Lewis, isn't it? Your case is still waiting to be considered."

"Still? WAITING? To be ***considered?*** What in hell *is* this? I've been in this Big rotten-Apple city for a YEAR and my case is still on the *WAITING LIST?"*

Shrug again. "Says so here."

"Ma'am." I stabbed the air with one index finger. If she were a man, I'd have emphasized each word with a poke on the chest. "If you people's paychecks rode on your ability to settle a case, you'd have completed mine long ago. Or been fired. In my entire life I have never had to deal with such an irresponsible, slow agency."

I am flying off the handle — God, was that shrink in Oregon right? Well, I'm steamed up and I can't put on the brakes now, so I plunge onward. "You call yourselves public servants, but you give service to no one. You're like college kids showing up for class just to catch a nap and get the credits, except you show up for coffee klatsch and paychecks. You are like the Three Wise Monkeys, except your names are Know Nothing, Do Nothing, Think Nothing. Your Do Nothing work mode destroys people's lives — and you just ... don't ... CARE."

It was April, 1985. We hit the road for Seattle, I driving a Plymouth Duster with a U-Haul in tow, Tina driving her Pinto, both of us equipped with CB radios so we could communicate while we were on the move, and Andrea having a wonderful trip bouncing back and forth from car to car.

No one in Tina's family could understand why we were moving. It simply would not register with them that we deplored the city lifestyle; they could not comprehend what we meant by being free to do what we liked without being suspicious of everyone and everything around us.

Five days and three thousand miles later we arrived in Kent, Washington, on the outskirts of Seattle.

11

We hit town early in the morning and spent the day resting up at my mom's. The next day we moved into the apartment that awaited us. Our own place at last: a palace of a place in a complex boasting a pool, hot tub, weight room, and honest to God parking — our own parking stalls, right beside our door. For $250 a month we had what would have cost at least a grand in New York.

The second day back home — *Home! Puget Sound in the spring!* — I went into the Seattle VA Regional Office and informed them of my change of address, and asked them to follow up on my request to have my records transferred from New York.

Voice On My Shoulder snickered. *What, no confidence in the Apple City office's ability to get the job done?* I told Voice I didn't have a speck.

I called my Green River Community College classmate and best friend, Ted, to announce my return the neighborhood. Part of my success at GRCC I owe to Ted; when the Crohn's flared up and I was unable to attend classes, Ted brought my assignments to the house and tutored me in lost lessons. The pair of us spent many a weekend fishing, gold panning, walking the hills ... things I hoped my little daughter would be doing with me in a year or three.

Amid all the wonder, Tina, Andrea, and I just turned 'round and 'round, wrapping ourselves in the beauty of home. Over there, Mt. Rainier looming through the easterly clouds; turn around and feast on the rainforested Olympic Mountains standing sentinel across sparkling Puget Sound; and all around and over us, clear, colorless, sea-freshened air you dare to inhale.

While I was still in New York I had contacted the few lighting firms in Washington. Now it was time to follow through.

Bottom line: Within three weeks I was at work in Seattle. South Seattle. Only a twenty-minute drive up Interstate 5.

I would be designing custom lighting fixtures. My new company dealt in one-of-a-kind custom fixtures for commercial clients — motels, restaurants, casinos, and the occasional individual willing to pay our price for specially designed arrangements. I reveled in the unfettered imagination allowed me, as long as I remained within the basic parameters of the job request. It was Alex in New York who taught me the trade; but it was Jim in Seattle who tossed out the challenges.

My biggest challenge was choosing from the vast array of materials I had to work with. In Alex's stock-lighting shop we used a basic sheetmetal fixture with a glass lens. In this custom work we used highly polished metals, wood, glass, acrylics. Instead of five to ten pound fixtures measured in inches, I now crafted artistic structures weighing hundreds, a thousand pounds, measured by the foot. My engineering studies really paid off here, even if I didn't ace the classes. I was amazed I retained so much; I even knew the concepts I blew in college. Obviously, real-life applications make things come together.

I was on the job a month and a half when the Crohn's disease really kicked my ass. I couldn't stand straight, could scarcely walk, and all my strength seemed to evaporate.

The Seattle VA wasn't interested in providing any assistance because the disease still was not service connected. It wouldn't have mattered anyway, because my records, which might justify my eligibility, had not arrived from New York.

Jim realized I had something serious, but once again I couldn't let a boss know it was Crohn's. Jim did know I should have been under the VA's assistance and that the VA wouldn't do anything; so he jockeyed my employment date so I was eligible for company insurance.

Without insurance, the cost of a doctor's care, tests, and probable hospitalization were simply wholly beyond my means, so while waiting for the policy to kick in I treated myself at home. But it was a horror cycle: without proper treatment it would take me longer to recover, and thus keep me away from work longer. I thought it wasn't possible for my condition to worsen, but it did. I ended up going to a doctor my mother referred me to.

The doctor, an internist, wanted to gurney me into the hospital immediately.

I decided to be level and upfront. "I can't do that. My previous employer's health insurer refused to cover me for the Crohn's problem because it was considered a chronic pre-existing condition," I said. "I won't jeopardize myself again by having a hospital admission on my record."

And isn't it interesting how the insurance companies relate the Crohn's to my military service but the VA can't find a connection.

"Well, it looks like Crohn's disease to me, and right now you are having a serious exacerbation of it," the doc said. "But you need to get stabilized before we can run the test. This prescription will relieve some of the pain. Bedrest, liquids only — you obviously know the routine."

I was too sick for much of anything *but* bedrest, but I didn't rest very well. With my design table set up I worked when I was able, which was precious little. I was in horrible, awful, bad shape ... I should have agreed with the doctor and checked myself into the hospital ... real bad shape.

I called the VA. If only I could find a VA doctor to examine me while I was in this condition . . .

"Mmm," said the Voice Of The VA, as if trying to fool me into thinking it was actually thinking. "Nothing here indicating you have any service related digestive disorder. Crohn's, you say? I don't see the word — "

"That is my very point. I *do* have Crohn's disease and the VA denies it is service connected because the VA doctors gave me an improper physical at the very outset. Now, because of a VA doctor's error, the VA apparently isn't willing to talk about it again, ever. Now I am in the midst of a major attack, and if you would admit me and conduct a proper diagnosis it would be obvious."

"Mmm," it said again, as if trying to fake thinking for the second time in the same day. "Well, there's nothing here to show you're entitled to be treated at a VA facility for whatever it is that's bothering you."

Just then a white-hot nova of pain exploded inside me and knocked the wind out of me and I doubled over. This was happening three, four times a day now: pain so unbearable, at times I wished I was dead.

"Six years," I gasped.

"Hmm?"

"It's been six years" ... inhale ... "and the VA has not even" ... exhale ... "once" ... gasp ... "tried to resolve this problem."

"Mmm, Mr. Lewis, you sound like you should get yourself to a doctor."

Well, it sure was obvious that the person behind the voice met the VA's strictest requirement for employment: It had a Moron Factor of 2.

The bottom line about the hospital issue is that I was scared of bankruptcy. If a person doesn't have a superlative insurance plan they are screwed. Even if I had a good one, the company could balk about pre-existing condition and stick me with the bill. I advocate socialized medicine if that's what it would take so that every man, woman, and child can see a doctor or even be hospitalized. No one should ever be denied proper medical care because of the status of his finances.

I was finally able to return to work on a regular schedule. I spent a hell of a lot of time in the men's room, and I could feel the boss's aggravation over that. Eventually he asked me about it and it was time, at last, to tell him I had Crohn's disease.

"Well, that's a relief," Jim smiled. "I thought maybe you had cancer."

I explained Crohn's disease, and although I am sure he understood the rudiments, I sensed he had a problem dealing with it. I didn't have time to worry about what he thought, however, because I was backlogged with work. We were swinging into our high season of production, with orders coming in every day.

The same weekend I moved my family from the apartment to a house — a real house with a yard of our own — Bob Finkleman moved from Klamath Falls to Seattle. One of the friends who helped stage the infamous anniversary disaster, who led me to the counseling group, fellow student at OIT, single guy, Bob had just completed his degree in drafting and was more than ready to go to work ... he had his student loan to pay off.

Only that week I had mentioned to Jim that I was swamped with new orders and I really needed some help. "A college classmate of mine just got his degree in drafting," I said, "and I would sure recommend him as our man."

I gave Bob's phone number to Jim. The two met, mutually interviewed one another, and Bob immediately became the firm's newest employee.

Bob was a fine draftsman and I educated him about the lighting industry as we went along. I made the basic design work-ups, and Bob composed the detailed drawings and blueprints for the production department. Together, we generated the kind of synergy in which one and one equaled more than two.

Increasingly, I worked with the shop crew, showing them different and more efficient techniques. Jim assigned me to research and develop two new projects. Not so gradually at all, I assumed more and greater responsibilities and I didn't mind that a bit; I loved the lighting business, loved my work.

I had never really recovered from my last Crohn's episode. I used more sick days than when I worked for Alex (which, in an unspoken way, Jim let me know displeased him), and when I was at work, I spent a good chunk of my time in the bathroom. I had frequent meetings with clients, and I was constantly terrified of having an accident. As a result, I was not eating properly — hell, I scarcely ate at all — and the lack of proper nutrition left me tired, sleepy, and unenergetic. All that had an obvious effect on my performance at work.

Jim, owner of the company, boss-man, a quick study (he was a fisherman by profession but he learned lighting quickly), and generally nice guy, was also a golf fanatic. Far too often, he bopped into my office, insisting I drop everything, no matter my workload or degree of concentration, to knock out eighteen holes. His golfing started standing in the way of deadlines, and he was quite willing to be late with a job, or expect the shop labor to make up for the time I lost on a project while golfing with the boss. When clients complained, I had to be the man to fabricate the excuses because, in the last analysis, I was the one responsible for getting the job done.

Jim also had a pathological, anti-social habit. He came to work with a predetermined decision to pick on a particular person that day. All day. Nobody could find any reason for his choice of victim of the day; it was as if he drew a name from a hat. No one was exempt; the hat also contained the name of his own daughter, who was our secretary. Then he rode the hell out of the unlucky one for the entire day.

His favorite tactic was sneaking up on his day's target and launching a tirade and scaring hell out of the recipient of his little game. In a manufacturing shop with all that power equipment and tools, it was a dangerous thing to do.

One day while I was on my forced ride to the links with him, Jim started bragging about how he got off on crawling his employees. He opened the door and I gladly stepped through.

"That's a lousy way to establish rapport and relationships, and a childish, asinine way to show leadership and managership," I told him. "Besides, the company owner hasn't any business in the shop; that's why you have supervisory personnel, and you are undermining them."

"Oh, shit, Chuck, I just kid around for fun. Besides, I am the BOSS and I sign the paychecks and anyone doesn't like a paycheck can leave."

"Being harassed isn't particularly fun. In my opinion management by intimidation is not a healthy practice. Stifling your employees' productivity costs you money, are you too dim to see that? Hell, we're up to our asses in a swamp and the gators are snapping, Jim. Besides that, with the workload we have, there just isn't time for that kind of bullshit conduct from the boss. For that matter, there isn't time to run around clobbering golf balls, either."

A muscle twitched in my boss's jaw. His eyes stared straight ahead.

"I'll tell you something else you urgently need to know," I continued. "I have Post Traumatic Stress Disorder. Shrink-signed and certified. You will be putting yourself at serious risk if you ever sneak up behind me and go into one of your screaming tirades. I would react to you the same as I'd react to any Gook who snuck up behind me, automatically and without a prior plan. I am very subject to jumping into the middle of your chest while I try to rip your head off."

"PTSD. I understand what you're talking about," Jim said quietly. "My son-in-law is a Nam vet. He goes into those raging reactions to loud noises, aggressive motions, to being startled. Hard to live with. Sometimes it's kind of scary to be around him."

"Well, you're just the onlooker, and if it scares you, imagine how *he* feels when this uncontrollable monster suddenly wakes up and takes over and he knows he can't stop it."

Jim nodded, looking a bit stricken. "Never though of it that way."

"Well, here's something else to think about, Boss. Our country is well populated with vets having stress syndrome of one degree or another. From World War Two, Korea, Nam, and whatever little 'Peace Keeping' wars the bureaucrats decide to send Americans to. You don't know who they are and you don't know what aggressive or insulting little thing is going to set them off, so the best thing everybody in this country can do is to keep their tongues still and their hands to themselves."

I inclined my head toward my boss. "Including you, Jim. You have three vets from the Korean War and four from Nam in that shop, and from your so-called kidding around, I'm real amazed you haven't had your lights punched out many times over."

"Hey, Chuck? You want to talk to my son-in-law? You know ... let him meet someone who understands?"

"Hell, I'll do better than that. There's a pretty good PTSD counseling service at the local vet center. I'd be proud to take him to the sessions. And, Jim, you're right: A man really does need to talk with someone who understands."

Jim maneuvered into a parking stall in front of the clubhouse but didn't switch off the ignition. "So ... you ready for some golf or what?"

I met his gaze and raised my eyebrows but didn't say a word.

"Yeah. Me, neither," he said, putting the car in gear and backing out. "Let's get back to the shop and knock out some work."

We rode to the office in silence but inside I smiled and hummed. I had just seen my boss and friend through two turning points. God, I like this job.

12

This is a record of my "progress" with the Veterans Administration of the United States of America since my discharge from the U.S. Army four years ago.

• Six visits to VA regional offices to review my claim.
• Four annual physical evaluations, required to keep disability awards up-to-date and continuing.
• Approximately three dozen phone calls to various offices and departments, most of which were responded to with the answer, "Gee, I don't know."
• One appeal (filed twice) theoretically in progress, but which whereabouts my local office claims not to know.

For the required physical check-up, each year I fill out the same-old forms from scratch, re-describing my medical problems. *Yeah, they pitch it out after each visit.. No use keepin' all that paper 'round the office, Miss Mellow.*

Each time, I include Crohn's disease as a service-related condition and each time I re-request a medical doctor's evaluation for it. Each time, the VA ignores it. The VA orders doctors to examine me only for the problems already cited on my record. Therefore, says the VA, since the word Crohn's is not on my record I do not have it. *Wonda wonda! S'poze we could get the VA to make poverty, crime, and illiteracy go away, too?*

This is excerpted from the official document the VA Regional Office sent the VA Medical Center; it is the VA's instructions to the physician:

02 AUG 83
REQUEST FOR PHYSICAL

Examination Limited To Disabilities Checked in Item 13, and/or listed in Item 14

ITEM 13: (check disabilities for which exam is needed)

— Foot injury
— Back injury
— Hearing loss

ITEM 14: Other Disabilities (List diagnosis or symptoms for which exam is requested)

(NOTHING ENTERED)

So there I had it. Now I knew why all my attending physicians said they could not evaluate me for Crohn's disease — because the VA told them they couldn't. They were explicitly to ignore any point that was not on the formal request. The doctors were just following instructions.

This is how (wave the banner) Our Government (roll the drums) takes care of its veterans? What low-rung bureaucrat at the Regional Office has a license to decree what is a medical problem and what is not? Yet the clerk can dictate to the doctors what they can and can not evaluate, and the doctors' hands are tied, regardless of any other conditions they observe.

Finally now, I understand the hostility I witnessed at that veterans' meeting in New York. Now I understand one more reason for the climbing suicide rate among Vietnam vets.

And suddenly I understood something else, too: Vietnam cost this country much more than it expected, thanks to new medical technologies. With Air-Evac helicopters, the wounded were moved to hospitals in a matter of minutes, and the hospitals had major new techniques in use. This created an extremely high survival rate, a rate which brought home many more men than our government had expected to have to care for, wounded and disabled as so many survivors were. In other words, more of us were supposed to die and thus eliminate the need to draw so heavily from the VA's budget.

So the government, a.k.a. the Senate and the House of Representatives and theoretically guided and goaded by the President, has a dilemma. Does it cheat people out of legitimate claims so it can stay within its budget? The system — the national legislature and all its agencies — has made it easy to ignore, or procrastinate to death, the cases and claims of veterans who have no other place to go for help.

As a result, most 'Nam veterans have done, or eventually will do, one or more of the following:

(1) Get totally frustrated and quit dealing with the VA entirely.

(2) Give up on everything, including life itself, because they can no longer bear the pain and agony and a nothingness future.

(3) Turn to drugs or alcohol, resulting in broken families, joblessness, homelessness, or permanent homes in prison. The government winds up spending more on them than the VA would have spent by fixing the problem in the first place.

(4) Not quit, continue to fight for what is rightly theirs, carry the torch for others who can't or won't fight for themselves. These are among the very few.

Now, a generation later, the aftermath of Vietnam is still with us. The loosening of morals, loveless lovemaking, children without marriage. The defiance of rules and order which arose from the protestations of our involvement in Southeast Asia in the first place. The ensuing disrespect for government leaders and the military establishment. The abandonment of veterans in need, resulting in broken marriages, broken families, children deserted and in poverty. Court systems which only dispense punishment when frustrated veterans finally break down.

All right, so Korean War veterans are old geezers now, and Vietnam vets are getting there. So the problem will go away in twenty, twenty-five years, right? Wrong. Our government has sent and will continue to send the next two generations of youngsters on "police actions" and "peacekeeping missions" to ... pick a continent; hell, if you're in the National Guard, pick a U.S. city.

And officially, there will be no such thing as Gulf War Syndrome, no Bosnia Crud, there is no malaria in the tropics, and L.A. sniper bullets are only imaginary.

13

In August 1985 Tina took a job installing temporary wall partitions in large office complexes. We enrolled four-year-old Andrea in preschool. At last we had two jobs and a decent income. In addition, Bob rented a room in the house and also helped out with household expenses. I thought we were finally getting our lives together.

I thought wrong. All of a sudden Tina didn't have time for me or our daughter. The same old crap started all over again, Tina wanting to live as if she were free, single, and monied. She attended parties which she meticulously engineered me out of. Despite our two incomes we still had nothing, and I had no idea where our cash was flowing.

All right, Tina had a right to be frustrated. My Crohn's disease effected our social life, but it didn't eliminate it if I was careful. But I thought Tina understood it's the disease that controls, not I.

Tina began to "have to" go to the local pubs with the guys after work, then "forget" to pick up Andrea at afterschool daycare. Many a time, someone at daycare called me at work in Seattle, asking me to come pick Andrea up because her mother had not.

Tina's occasional bouts became a consistent habit and it was a financial drain in three ways: The money she drank up, the extra fees for extended day care, and the time I had to take from work to care for Andrea. I had no idea how much Tina earned because she never showed me a pay stub, nor did she ever make a deposit in our bank account.

I couldn't carry the rent plus all the other costs of living, and Tina never contributed to the household. So in November we moved. Again. But, oh well ... we were so far behind in the rent we were about to be evicted anyway. Why, with the two of us earning a paycheck, were we always broke before the next payday?

Tina wanted to go into Seattle for a weekend cultural fest. "Andrea would enjoy seeing the people and the sights. So would you. You need to lighten up, take some recreational time, Chuck," she said, trying to make it into a family event instead of one for herself.

"I can't do it, Hon," I said. I was in the midst of another Crohn's episode and needed to catch up on missed work. Tina knew that, of course.

"Well, okay, I'll ask Bob to take me."

"That's fine with me. The three of you have a good time."

"Well, I don't think Andrea would enjoy it. You keep her with you."

So ... She's going with Bob instead of me, and all of a sudden her daughter is excess weight!

At ten in the morning, as Tina hopped into Bob's car, she waved cheerfully. "Be back around six," she called.

At two in the morning they came stumbling in about half crocked. I would have put a hundred dollars on the table saying she was messing around on me, but I hadn't a bit of proof so I just took a watchful attitude.

Just before the Christmas holiday season began, Tina lost her job. Again. This time it was because of "a personality clash between me and the people at work. Besides," she said haughtily, "I'm just too educated to have to be forced to deal with the morons I work with."

What education? Tina had a GED. She talked the talk about college classes, but she had failed a majority of her classes and never completed any course or program.

"Besides, Chuck, if you had a reasonable-paying job you could support us decently, and I wouldn't *have* to work. I could devote myself to my daughter, and host parties to elevate *you* in *your* field."

Devote herself to her daughter ... as in yelling and slapping her around? Elevate *me* ? As in ignoring me in favor of drinking with the guys she works with? Support us? What happened to our agreement before I left the Army?

Actually I was quite satisfied with the $350 a week I took home, plus the $300 per month in disability comp from the VA.

What in the hell was her bitch, and where did her income go when she did work?

At work we were swamped with orders. We needed additional help. Since Ted had just been terminated in a "downsizing" of the firm he worked for, I recommended him to Jim. Ted was immediately taken on board, and what an asset he proved to be! He had a natural ability to make maximum use of materials available, doing things others thought impossible with shop machines and tools others didn't know how to utilize. While he was in school, his wife had given him a bunch of grief about not being in the workforce, so he didn't get to finish his drafting degree. I really could have used him in the design department, but Jim insisted he was only qualified for the shop.

Apparently Jim took seriously my little sermon about harassing employees, because he began knocking himself out being charitable and considerate. He got a half-dozen season tickets for his hero team, the Seattle Seahawks, and allowed employees to use them. He entered several of his employees in a golf tournament and paid the bill. He sponsored a company golf tournament, which he "selected" me to organize.

I accepted the "appointment," but reluctantly. I was more than usually engrossed in my work, and I really didn't need one more chore. On the other hand, it might be a welcome respite from Tina's crap at home; indeed, maybe work was so compelling because I no longer wanted to be home. I seriously thought of divorce.

On the surface, it was about money. Deeper, it was about a woman turned completely self-centered. Nothing was good enough for her; she constantly wanted more, more, more. She ruled out going back to work and she was unwilling (or not clever or selfless enough) to live within a single income. "If you can't earn enough to provide a high standard of living," she told me more than once, "you should get another job."

Just after Thanksgiving we moved — again — to a nice apartment in Auburn, just a couple of miles from Kent. Now it was time to prepare for Christmas. Again this year, Tina spent everything we had on gifts for her relatives — all her uncles, nephews, her five siblings. Was Tina so worried about looking good to her family that she was willing to have her own daughter go without?

I did what I hated: I hid money from Tina so I could get her and Andrea something for Christmas. I just couldn't make Tina understand that our obligations to each other and to our daughter were supposed to supersede whatever ones she felt she owed her family. She had no comprehension of her vow to "forsake all others." She apparently needed to create the illusion that we were better off than we were, and in doing that, she was putting herself in an ever increasing fantasy world. Each time I felt I was stepping up, Tina wanted more. I finally figured out that I would never be able to satisfy her.

For some time now, Jim had been accepting job contracts for which we couldn't possibly meet promised delivery dates. He made major design changes without clients' knowledge. We were up to our asses in work and getting more and more backlogged. We desperately needed more people, but the only word Jim could think of was "layoffs." Here we were, oversold and understaffed, and all Jim said was, "Anyone who can't stand the pressure can walk."

In an effort to finish more projects faster, Jim decided to allow some of the not-so-qualified to take over projects. For a client, I designed a fixture that called for Plexiglas rods to hang through a sheet of Plexiglas, with lights in the center. The rods were of varied lengths, creating a pattern. The rods passed through the plex base, eliminating the need to use ugly fastening devices, while also allowing the fixture to be serviced without having to screw the rods apart. (There were about a hundred rods in this fixture. Can you imagine having to unscrew every rod to clean the fixture or replace lamps?) The client approved my design, and that was he expected to get.

The young apprentice assigned to assemble the fixture didn't understand what I wanted to do with the rods. Instead of asking me, he sat on the job trying to figure things out for himself.

Bob happened to be working behind a partition in the shop when Jim came in and jumped on the fellow. "How can you be so darn slow on such a darn simple fixture!" Jim bellowed.

"I'm trying to figure out what Lewis wants done here," the intern explained.

"Why didn't you go ask?" Jim demanded.

"Because," the frustrated youngster wailed. "If he thinks I'm too stupid to figure things out he'll never recommend me for promotion to journeyman!"

"Hey. Forget Lewis. Go ahead and do it the old way. Let's just get this damn job done and out of here."

The "old way" changed the number of parts, the method of assembly, invalidated my assembly instructions, and altered the product the client thought he was getting. Puzzled and perplexed with the changes in assembly, the youngster lost track of what he was doing. He spent two or three days bumbling with the assembly, falling even farther behind. Finally Jim paid him a stomping-hollering visit.

"I want that sorry fixture shipped out *now!*" he stormed. "The client's raising hell about this mess being so late. Send it out now!"

"It isn't quite done yet," said the cadet.

"Send it out *now*!" Jim ordered.

Three days later I was twenty fathoms deep in concentration over a design for a large motel chain, while across the room Bob labored over his own thing. He works so quietly you scarcely notice he's there, which is one thing I like about him. There was a sudden roar and eruption behind me. Startled, I jumped, tearing my design. I spun around and grabbed Jim by the shirt collar and damn near took his head off. Shocking myself by my action, I let him go. "Jesus, Jim. Damn, I'm sorry. But gods, man, I warned you about doing that."

But my boss was only getting warmed up. "That fixture with the plex rods was all screwed up, and it was all your fault," Jim yelled.

"Far as I know, the job went according to blueprint. Nobody brought any problems to me," I said, puzzled. But Jim didn't hear me because he was still yelling.

I walked away, leaving him screaming in my office, and went to the shop to talk with the apprentice. There I discovered what happened—at least *his* view of the story.

I returned to my office and called the contractor who was trying to install the fixture. He described the problems he was having. What happened was that Jim had redesigned the fixture but not the installation instructions. Furthermore, the package was shipped incomplete; parts had been made but not shipped.

I arranged to ship the missing pieces and promised the contractor I'd rewrite the instructions. Then I went to have some words with Jim.

I collected my composure as best I could, but I was so angry I shook. I was a basket case of raw nerves; Jim may never realize how close he came to being taken out permanently. I was not about to be his little target for the day just because he interfered with what would have been a first-class product for a client.

"In the future," I told Jim, "you are to inform me when you make changes to my designs. You will not make *me* responsible for screw-ups caused by changes *you* make. Is that clear?"

Jim's eyes widened and he whimpered a little as he nodded, but I didn't let him get a word in. "I apologize for grabbing you," I said. "But I told you before about the danger you'd be in if you snuck up behind me and went into one of your fits. And now," I said, opening to door to his office and stepping through it, "I have to go take a walk."

For an hour and a half I wandered the local neighborhood and at noon I went to a restaurant where guys in the shop often had lunch. Ted came in and joined me.

"Jim wants me to get the keys to your office," Ted said, intently watching himself stir, stir, stir his coffee. "I'm supposed to tell you not to go back to work."

"He appointed you as hatchet man? To tell me I'm fired?"

Ted kept stirring.

"Listen, Ted. I have no problem accepting responsibility for my mistakes, but I refuse to accept responsibility for someone else's. There are standards of conduct, lines that even the owner of a business is not allowed to cross. Jim took massive leaps over those lines."

I gave Ted my keys. "You can pick me up here after work," I told him. We were carpooling to work and this was his day to drive.

I told Ted I'd need to get to the office to pick up my tools and designing equipment. We agreed that I would go with him on Saturday, when he went in to finish his current project.

I had developed a pretty good reputation within the custom lighting industry. Finding another job would be no problem. The problem would be explaining things to Tina.

Tina's eyes widened and darkened. "It's your fault! Your own freaking idiot fault! Can't just do things the way they've always been done, have to get artsy-fartsy smartsy, screw it up —"

Ted broke in. "It wasn't Chuck's screw-up, Tina." I had asked Ted to stand by while I talked to Tina and I was glad now for his support. "Jim's the one who messed up," Ted tried to explain.

Tina kept wringing her hands and crying. "How are we going to get by? Why can't you be a provider? What am I going to do?"

What was *she* going to do?

I didn't feel like making an issue of the incredible self-centeredness of that remark, so I let it go. Instead, I said, "Listen, Hon. We aren't destitute yet. I have a couple of thousand put aside, and that will tie us over until I get another job. I have a lot of contacts and some damn good references."

Tina quit sobbing and started screeching. "Two thousand! You hoard money and then turn around and tell me we couldn't afford to get Christmas presents for my sisters and nieces and nephews? You tell me I can't have the things I want, and you have *two grand* hidden away? What kind of provider *are* you, anyway?"

Ted had already slipped away. I decided to get out of there, too. Here I thought it was so great that I could tell my wife we had the financial wherewithal to sustain ourselves for two or three months. Then, instead of being grateful for the stash, she was angry I had it. I was really starting to wonder if Tina's head was screwed on right.

The job search began. I went to people I had done jobs for in the past. I traveled all over Washington and Oregon, inquiring of every architectural design firm. All with the same results. "We aren't hiring at this time," or, "We are already overstaffed," or, "The costs of insurance and fringes make it prohibitive to take on more employees."

Ted dropped by one afternoon while I was scrubbing the kitchen floor. "Sit," Ted ordered. I sat.

"I heard some of those 'Joe told Mac that Arthur told him' conversations in the locker room," Ted said, handing me a can from the six-pack of soda he had brought. "Jim's been bragging that he set up that light-fixture incident in order to get rid of you, Chuck. A guy in the shop mentioned that Jim said he's, quote, tired of having to put up with that Crohn's disease smokescreen, but he knew he'd have to set something up where, quote, Lewis couldn't nail Jim for discrimination. Jim rigged up the situation so he could fire you for misconduct, Chuck, and now he's gleeful because that makes you are ineligible to draw unemployment."

I carried this information to the employment office and demanded a hearing.

Ted's testimony was not taken because he had heard everything second hand, so it was unallowable.

Not one person spoke up on my behalf. They all corroborated Jim's assertion of my misconduct. Even Bob, my so-called long time friend from college, who helped me with the entire project, who worked right next to me when Jim made the scene in the office the one who saw and heard so much of it first-hand. He told the hearing examiner he witnessed none of it. I reminded myself that these former friends and associates weren't just thinking of their own skins; they had families, siblings, children, elderly parents. Each man was responsible for a whole sphere of others. I don't know, maybe I wouldn't have jeopardized my wife and baby and livelihood for one of them, either.

Ted told me that customers were abandoning Jim's ship like lemmings jumping off a cliff. A slew of Jim's former clients asked me to consider setting up my own company. "We'll bring our business to you," they promised me. I had assurances of a future business and I had explicit, concrete job orders awaiting. Ted not only encouraged me, he set out helping me investigate sources for start-up funding. We agreed to make it a business partnership. Ted would be a loyal friend and a trusted associate.

We spent the summer and fall investigating every avenue to obtain the necessary start-up funding. Nowhere. Not the VA; it didn't extend small business loans to Vietnam vets. Not the Small Business Administration, which was happy to enroll me in its classes but "unable" to float me a start-up loan. For me, part of The American Dream, the one where a person launches his own business, fizzled out.

All the while, the best Tina could do was sit around and bitch because I didn't have a job. She was completely unsupportive about my starting my own business and she didn't give a rip whether I did or not. The only thing she knew was that is wasn't supposed to be her responsibility to find a job. That was my duty.

By late fall all my avenues were exhausted and so were our finances. Again unable to swing the rent, we moved back in with my folks.

14

By now I couldn't hide my condition from any potential employer. Job applications ask about medical problems. I had to answer truthfully because the disease kept flaring up and causing complications and grief, just as it had with Jim. I heard all excuses known to man for not being hired. Hopelessness thrived in me. More and more, the VA's failure to deal with my case critically effected my life.

Crowded into my parents' two-bedroom apartment, we were as close to homeless as a family can get and still be out of the elements. My VA disability check of $389 a month couldn't feed and house us, I couldn't get a loan to start up the business that was guaranteed to prosper and I couldn't get a job, and Tina refused to even try.

Finally, as a last resort, Mom and Dad helped us move into an apartment in Pacific. The place was a real dump, a fire waiting to happen, and the landlord reminded me of the birds of prey we left back in New York. But it made us eligible for assistance from welfare. That supplemented my disability payments by an additional $113 a month, plus $35 more in food stamps, and now, for the first time since I had been discharged from the Army, I had medical care available to me. We sure wouldn't be living the good life, but with care we could make it from payday to payday ... if Tina could put a brake on her selfish impulse spending.

That was the year Andrea started kindergarten. I hated sending my baby to school dressed in the tatters she had, but we had no money for better.

All the evidence made it look as if Tina deliberately set out to discourage, to run me down. Where she could have leveled with her folks, probably gotten them to at least buy some decent clothes for their granddaughter, she lied. I heard her phone conversations — long-distance calls we couldn't afford.

"Things are really rosy, couldn't be going greater," she kept telling them. "Chuck is making big money, we'll be owning our own company in a short time." Then she'd pour it on about her social and cultural life, even making up a couple of snobbish civic "committees" to put herself on.

The only thing she said that was remotely true was that the VA still hadn't done a damn thing, and that the Crohn's was controlling my life even more.

Heavy duty hopelessness set in, and a sense of helplessness; God, I felt so helpless. And alone, so damned alone. I had no understanding person to talk to. I felt I had lost control of everything in my life. A running thread in my thoughts was . . . doing myself in. Tina and Andrea could get on with their lives without me to hinder or hold them back.

Again, I contacted the VA to try to find out what was happening with my claim. All I got was the same old line. Finally I did what I should have thought of long ago but didn't: I called my congressman.

I went to Congressman Elliott's local office and filed a complaint against the VA, giving his staff all the pertinent information. "We'll do everything possible to help you," the staffer assured me. "But it may take some time to get all the information processed and the case resolved."

"What's new?" I quipped.

"Finally, some action," I told myself as I drove to the dump I called home. "I hope The Congressman From The Great State Of Washington rips them apart."

In Kent I found a doctor who specialized in inflammatory bowel disease. Thank God for the medical coupons from welfare.

Dr. Fien took the entire medical history of my Crohn's problem — the first person to ever do so. "My opinion is that you do indeed have Crohn's disease," he said, "but we need to run some tests to confirm it."

Here was a doctor who, based on my medical history, concluded I had some sort of digestive disorder, and he did it within the first few minutes of my first visit. Yet the VA never considered running even the first diagnostic test. A strange feeling swept over me that the VA intentionally attempted to sabotage my claim.

I underwent the workups necessary for a proper diagnosis. Dr. Fien took three entire appointments to run the tests the VA claimed were not needed.

First, the sigmoidoscopy, the insertion of a fiber-optic scope into the rectum, to examine the large intestine. Despite the sedative he gave me, the pain was awesome, but it ruled out ulcerative colitis.

Next, the barium enema. That was a whole new definition of pain ... and pain. Three days on my back and a week of lingering hurt. But it established the probability of Crohn's.

Finally, the Upper GI (gastro intestinal) series of tests. They came out positive for Crohn's and pinpointed the site of the problem.

Tina and I went together to the doctor's office to discuss the disease and my future with it. This Dr. Fien made clear: There is no cure for Crohn's disease. Its cause is unknown. Those facts I already knew from my own research. The doctor told us that in some cases, surgery is necessary and can lessen some of the symptoms and alleviate the pain; but surgery does not constitute a cure, because the disease reasserts itself about a year after the diseased section of the intestine is removed. My Crohn's would in time get worse, but there was no way to predict how much worse, since it effects different patients in different ways, to different degrees.

"Sounds like I have one hell of a future to look forward to."

The doctor nodded but Tina's eyes had that flat, uncomprehending expression. *Strange ... before I got out of the service I didn't realize how dim that woman is. She just doesn't get things.*

Therefore, it was mostly for Tina's benefit that I said, "Okay, Dr. Fien, let's go over this whole program, make sure we know what I can expect." I grasped Tina's hand and squeezed—not as a gesture of affection but as a try at cutting through the fog—and told her, "Any questions you have, be sure to ask. This is your life, too, Hon."

"Well, what you're going to have, Mr. Lewis, is more or less constant pain and diarrhea ... for the rest of your life. It's possible you'll have to have portions of the intestines removed. If so, you'd have the burden of a colostomy bag."

"Explain what that entails." I had seen wounded men leaving hospitals at the front with colostomy bags, so I knew what that meant, but I wanted the doc to be the one to say it to Tina.

"It's an external bag attached to a hole in the abdomen. Bowel fluids drain into it."

"So it goes without saying that wearing a baggie is both uncomfortable and embarrassing," I said. "If nothing else it will surely cause a major slowdown in my lifestyle."

Dr. Fien nodded again. "Your diet will also have to undergo a radical change. Foods that are healthy are a no-no for you now. No fresh veggies, fruit with peels, nuts, garlic, milk products, no foods high in fiber."

When the doc asked her, Tina said yes, she understood. "Means our social life pretty much comes to a halt," she summed up.

Hear that, Lewis? Her priority isn't your health. The important thing to her is she won't have an escort who looks like the cover of a romance novel.

Dr. Fien gave us some reading material about the disease and information about the National Foundation for Ileitis and Colitis.

"Big favor to ask, Dr. Fien," I said. "Would you be willing to help me with my case with the VA?" I explained about the runaround game the VA was playing with me.

"That's a surprise, how the VA's service has obviously deteriorated since I was on staff at the VA hospital," the doctor said. "I'm pretty upset about how the agency has altogether neglected your complaint."

"You were a VA doctor?" It was my turn to be surprised. *I guess the good ones can't stand it and bail out.*

My next appointment was scheduled and I was sent on my way with a ton of drugs that were supposed to abate the pain and diarrhea. (Which they didn't.) The other medication Dr. Fien gave me was a permanent prescription for Prednisone.

Prednisone, he explained, is a cortisone based steroid. With some interesting side effects. Diabetes, glaucoma, cataracts; suppression of the immune system, increased sweating and the resultant foul body odor; mental or emotional disturbances, loss of bone strength causing spontaneous fractures; suppression of the body systems to the extent that a person on Prednisone can't go under general anesthesia.

And Prednisone has this neat little habit of attacking the brain; specifically it singles out the memory cells. Now that's just what I need — drug induced dementia. It's not bad enough to have to deal with Crohn's disease, but I get to take drugs that mess me up even more.

Rosy future, ha! I was better off not knowing what I was up against, just dealing with the pain and diarrhea on my own.

I was in a state of shock over the magnitude of the effect this disease had on me and the difficulty of adjusting to it. I saw my chances of leading a normal, productive life — what can I say? — go down the toilet.

I knew that Tina understood the implications of all this, too, because she gasped once, sighed twice, and her eyes swam. But for once in her life she listened without opinionating.

Once again my mind grasped at the thought: The only way I could acquire security and certainty of my future was to start my own business. There must be some avenue ... millions of people establish their own companies ... surely I can not be on the lowest rung of the ladder of competence ...

Officially, the VA offers financial assistance to veterans starting their own businesses — but only to vets of Korea and earlier. No business loans for vets of Nam, or Desert Storm, or the myriad of "peace police" "non-conflicts" to which the United States its defenders to be killed or maimed for no compensation. After Vietnam I remained in the Army; and with that modicum of insulation I remained ignorant of how America treated my returning brothers in arms. Most 'Nam vets returned home and from all external appearances they were productive, well-adjusted members of mainstream society — people in education, business, the professions, trades, the service sector . Many never discuss their military service; they hold it all inside. All too many of them also carry lingering psychological disorders, the effects of that war still haunting them.

On a late-night talk show in November, 1986 we saw a recruiting commercial for the Coast Guard. "There you go, Hon," I jested. "You join up, integrate the ranks in a way they never dreamed of, and I'll be your dependent."

"Yeah, right." She winked and grinned. "I bring in the payola and the check's got my name on it. So that makes me the head of the household and you have to do as I say!"

"I'll do anything you say, Baby!" I laughed. "And the USCG gets to furnish housing and pay the medical bills for your faithful dependent."

Tina must have semi-liked the idea of my dependency because took a holiday-season job at a toy store. Because she was only temporary part-time help, the money she made would not be deducted from our welfare assistance. I despised the welfare mindset that said don't do a thing to help yourself or you'll lose your payments; but now we were walking in those shoes and here we were, doing the same thing.

Tina's stated goal was to enable us to have a Christmas for Andrea. For Andrea? Ha! Andrea wound up getting a little two-dollar trinket from her mother, and once again Tina put on her Rich and Royal Act for her family. Spending every cent she earned on them. Keeping up the pretenses. Why could she not be honest with them? And still, after six years of her fakery, I didn't know how to do anything about it without creating more problems.

15

On the day before Christmas 1986 I received a letter from Congressman Elliott. Enclosed was a copy of a Notice of Disagreement which the Veterans Administration claimed it sent me. It stated, "Your claim ... has been denied. ... If you disagree with the current determination of your case you have sixty (60) days to respond in order to obtain further action."

Date of the latter: 18 October, 1982.

A Notice of Disagreement is the notification that a veteran's claim, or any part of a claim, has been denied. It explains the appeals procedure, and gives a claimant a time period in which to reply in order to contest the denial.

After reading and rereading it, I handed the papers to Tina. "Look at this," I fumed. "This is nothing short of a bunch of horse shit. For *FOUR YEARS* I have been penalized because I failed to respond to a document that I *NEVER GOT*."

That's right, I had never heard of a Notice of Disagreement and I had never received such a piece of paper.

With my index finger I stabbed the inside address printed on the letter. "Look at this. I never heard of it. This document was sent to a bogus address."

Now I was on a roll and gathering steam. I was thinking aloud, and for once Tina was being the ear I needed.

"Point number one is that I never saw this document." I picked up a dinette chair and plopped it down hard. *Good control, Lewis. You didn't break anything and you didn't smack anyone. Yet.*

"Point number two is a question. Is this the appeal that I am supposed to have in the works right now? The one I can't get any response about?

"Then, as a third point, there is this sixty day crock of crap."

Tina furrowed her brow, so I explained. "A veteran has one year from the most recent determination date to file an appeal. So where do they get off on this sixty day charade?

"And if you haven't gagged to death yet, there's point number four. If I don't notify them, the VA assumes all this is swell with me. Yet they have no way of knowing if I ever actually received this so-called Notice. So, for point number five, the VA drops life-or-death stuff like this in the mail, addressed to a nonexistent place, unregistered and uncertified, and assumes the veteran receives it. The United States Postal Service can't figure out that it should return an official-business, unclaimed letter sent to a noplace address. The VA depending on the Postal Service — Jesus, cross a nincompoop with an imbecile and what do you get?

A Statement of Case is a form which describes past decisions the VA has rendered in a veteran's case. It states the reasons for a decision, and it quotes pertinent laws and regulations. In short it provides all the hows and whys for a decision. A veteran must have this information in order to properly file an appeal, and by law the VA must provide it.

On December 29, 1986 I received from Congressman Elliott's office a copy of my Statement of Case. That document, too, was dated October 1982. By regulation, the Notice of Disagreement is supposed to go out first; then, if the vet chooses to appeal, the Statement of Case follows. I found it strange that both were dated the same day, and, presumably, allegedly sent to me in the same mailing.

This breach of procedure made it perfectly clear to me that the VA knew I intended to follow up on my claim — that they knew I would appeal it as far as necessary to get my entitlements. It looked to me like the VA purposely used a wrong address to delay my claim, giving themselves an easy excuse to dismiss the whole case because "the veteran failed to respond within the timely parameters designated."

I invited Ted over so I could vent on him. "This is a chicken shit a tactic if I ever saw one!" I railed, handing him both letters to eyeball. "Delay things for years and blame the delay on the veteran. Why in hell didn't at least one of those, capital letters-Our Public Servants, question why I didn't respond to the 1982 letters?" What I was looking at indicated that in four years not one of My Public Servants had even looked at my files.

Ted was always a good commiseration partner, and it happened that this time he needed an ear to vent into, too. So we drank a pot of coffee while Ted soothed me, then we switched to beer while I listened to him. Just before Christmas, Jim had fired Ted.

My personal theory: Jim figured out it was Ted who told me about Jim's setting things up to fire me. Jim had been pretty surprised when I told him I knew why I was fired and how he arranged it. Plus, after I was fired but while Ted still worked for Jim, Ted actively helped me in the hunt for start-up money for my business. We decided to enter into a business partnership: Ted would handle the shop, I'd manage the office. When (Not "if." "When.") the Crohn's flare-ups immobilized me, he'd be there to run the overall operation.

I have no doubt that Jim's antennae scoped out that information and used it against Ted.

In the end, the final laugh (in case anyone was laughing) was Jim's. I gave up on the going-into-business dream because I had exhausted all the possible resources I knew. Meanwhile, I continued the desperate search for work.

On the third of January 1987, Tina and I went into the Seattle Veterans Administration Regional Office to present my case, again, and to try to initiate some action, again. The office does not make appointments, so people try to arrive before sunup and come prepared to stay until dusk ... just like kids stake out campsites for a rock concert. It must be too simple for Our Public Servants to figure out that an appointment system would make it easier for all.

But, as Ted once said, then they'd have to think. Not to mention they might have to give up the coffee breaks between clients! If appointments were actually scheduled, they would have to see two vets in a row, back-to-back. That translates into work, and we can't have that now, can we?

Tina and I were the first to walk through the Regional Office door — the first clients of the new year.

We waited. For more than an hour.

We spent the time listening to the "service" reps joke and discuss their holidays as they had coffee klatsch. There were five performers (government employees) and five audience (clients waiting to be served). One would think these ignoramuses would have the common sense to at least go somewhere out of sight to not work. This must be what political candidates have in mind when they promise, "We will create jobs."

I had developed a bit of an attitude long before my name was finally called and Tina and I went to the designated cubicle.

Within a couple of minutes a clerk came in, coffee cup in hand. *Damn, this guy looks young! Fresh out of college, he looks. Too young to identify with problems of vets heading toward middle age.* He introduced himself and asked pleasantly, "And how may we help you today?"

"Well, the first way you could help is to maybe get me and my wife a cup of coffee. We've been waiting here so long our morning coffee has worn off."

"Oh, I'm sorry, I can't do that," he said pleasantly.

Okay, I sure can skip the pleasantries if you can. So I explained my case in outline form, just to get him thinking about his job.

Then I went through it all again, this time in great detail. Coming down with Chron's disease in the Army. The inexcusable excuse of a physical from the VA. The denial of service connection, medical insurance, and treatment, and the medical bills I incurred as a result. The appeal hearing that took place without my knowledge or presence, the denial of my right to present new evidence to support the appeal. The misaddressed Statement of Case and Notice of Disagreement dated October 1982, which, I explained, I received only last week and only through the efforts of my congressman.

I showed the youngster the Notice of Disagreement and the Statement of Case. "You can copy these and the rest of my file as well," I told him. "It would be helpful for you to have your own copy of everything I have."

All this telling, showing, explaining, and clarifying ate up an hour and some minutes. A very worthwhile hour, I figured. Wrong again!

The little VA kid leaned back in his cushioned roller-recliner-swivel chair and gazed at me expressionlessly. "So," he drawled, "Whatchya want me ta, y'know, do?"

Shocked, biting back quick-tempered, bitter retorts, I said the first neutral thing that popped into my mind. "You went to college?"

"Yeah," he grinned. "English lit. Summa cum laude."

"Well, Mr. Summa, I really would like to have my case reopened. That's what I came here for."

"I can reopen your claim, Mr. Lewis, but your *new* effective date will be today. That is to say, you cannot receive any *retroactive* benefits because your one-year time limit for filing an appeal expired three years ago. I can also tell you that your appeal will be denied right here and no further action will be taken."

"Wait a fucking minute here! You better give me a better answer than that."

"Mr. Lewis, your time to apply for another appeal of your claim expired in October of 1983. It is now January of 1987. I will admit that the "within 60 days" stipulation was in error; it should have stated "within one year." However, you did not follow up on your claim within the prescribed time period."

"Wrong answer, Mr. Summa. I received this letter only two weeks ago, and then it was only through the efforts, footwork, and sleuthing of my congressman. The way I see it, the effective deadline for filing an appeal has to be one year from the date I receive notification. Therefore, technically speaking, I am well within the prescribed time period. I received these documents on the twenty-fourth of December 1986. Anyone with anything more than jelly for brains can figure out that was less than a year ago."

"I'm sorry, Mr. Lewis . . ." *How can this kid remain so totally unmoved and practiced-polite? Doesn't he have an emotion chip?* ". . . but the fact remains that 1987 is not one year from 1982. Why you didn't receive the information the VA sent you is not the VA's problem. I can't do anything about it. Based on the fact that this case is so old, I can tell you that it will be denied without further action because you don't have enough evidence to support your claim here."

All the glue inside me popped loose. I jumped up on his desk and grabbed two hands full of the kid: collar, shirt, tie, jacket and all. I snatched him across the top of his desk, sending papers flying all over the floor. I yanked him up eyeball to eyeball with me as I explained a couple of the finer points of information to him.

"Let me tell you something, you snot nosed little shit. I have the right to file an appeal on all points of my case that I feel need to be addressed. I have cause to be reconsidered and I can not figure out why the only thing you can think of is excuses for why you shouldn't do what you are here to do."

My anger was feeding itself and I wanted to trash this whole cold uncaring cheating freaking rip-off place. I'd settle for taking out this insignificant arrogant little literature major instead. I shook the wimp again and I heard his eyeballs rattle. "Now where in the hell is your medical degree that you can diagnose my physical ailments? You are nothing but an entry-level processor of documents, and before I rip your pathetic head off your shoulders and piss down your bloody stump of a neck, you best get someone over here who knows what the hell they are here for. You sorry —"

Tina grabbed me.

I almost knocked her upside the head, but I didn't. I looked into her eyes and saw Andrea. I released the lit major and jammed my hands into my pockets. *My baby girl has her mother's eyes. My baby is going to be a beauty.* But it gave me great satisfaction to note the young snot-nosed entry-level clerk had turned white and he was immobile with fear.

Tina grasped my file in one hand and yanked at me with the other, dragging me toward the door. All the stuff on the kid's desk was all over the floor. Other employees stood around watching what was happening, but all kept their distance. Now I knew for sure that these people could not relate to veterans — can you imagine warriors in combat not aiding their brothers in arms? The concept of rescuing comrades is as foreign to these guys as the concept of life in another galaxy. *We have seen the enemy, and we tiptoed the hell away.*

After getting me into the hall and away from the target of my wrath, Tina convinced me to go have a cup of coffee and cool off while she looked up the local Disabled American Veterans organization. She'd find them, see if they could do anything to help. If so, she would set up an appointment with them. Then she'd meet me in the cafeteria.

I went to the basement of the Federal building, got coffee, and lowered myself to a heated boil.

Soon a couple of older guys took the table next to mine. They were talking about "the vet that just about trashed the VA office upstairs."

"It should happen more often," said one. "Maybe the VA would start taking veterans more seriously. Especially the Vietnam vets. The VA has been messing with them from the start, always changing the rules on them."

"Good thing that guy didn't get arrested," said the other. "I'd hate seeing a vet get arrested for standing up for his rights. Sure am glad the VA treated us World War Two vets better, but I keep hearing stories about how it's no longer a place to go for help. 'Specially for 'Nam vets."

The fellows seemed like comrades in mind, so I gathered the nerve to speak to them.

"I'm Chuck Lewis. The wacked-out vet you boys are talking about."

The pair wiggled a bit and looked down into their mugs. One began busying himself stirring coffee that had no sugar or cream to stir. I regretted embarrassing them.

I turned my chair to their table and sketched out my story, including the details of my "visit" to the office upstairs.

I was a paragraph or two from finishing my account when Tina arrived. I introduced her to the gentlemen, then wrapped up my story.

Then she said, "The DAV will see you this very day, Chuck."

"Yes, see them," the first gentleman said. "Those boys at DAV know the laws and regs, and they're good at representing vets' cases and claims to the VA."

"By all means see them," agreed the second. "Let them do your fighting for you. Then you have the power of an official veterans' organization backing you up. And you do have one hell of a case, you know."

"Thank you, guys. I'm beginning to realize getting my case completed involves a lot more than I first thought. I can see I definitely need some outside help if I'm ever going to get my entitlements from the VA."

I thanked my two new acquaintances for their insight and supportiveness. Then Tina and I headed out to see the DAV representative.

When you pay a call to any agency affiliated with veterans' service, the rigmarole is always the same. So I knew which order the hoops were to be jumped through: First fill out forms, the same ones you've filled out two or three or twenty-three times before, depending on how many times you've called on the agencies. Then sit and wait.

As I handed the completed form to the secretary, she asked cheerfully, "And are you a paid member of DAV?"

"No, not at this time. However, I was, several years ago."

"Surely you'd like to renew your membership?"

"I'll certainly consider that, provided the DAV does something to help me. They didn't do that before."

While I sat and waited for the rep to summon me, my mind churned over the events of the morning — man, it wasn't even noon yet! The old warriors in the cafeteria were right: I am damn lucky I didn't get hauled off to the slammer.

I was very scared of myself at that moment. I was afraid of going off the deep end and trashing out some poor dweeb who didn't know what he was doing. Does the VA make employees take the pledge to go out of their way to screw over a veteran?

After twenty minutes (a short wait by Federal standards) the DAV rep called me into his cubicle.

"Hello, I'm John and I'll be your DAV rep. Are you a paid-up member of DAV?"

Christ, don't these people worry about anything beyond paying up? "I hope membership is not a prerequisite for enlisting your help, because at this point I don't have ten dollars to join anything. The reason I haven't any extra tens is that I am a veteran who has been completely betrayed by the VA."

"No, membership isn't a requirement. Tell me about the VA."

So I told my story yet another time to still another listener. While I talked, John took notes. That was a heartening sign; that was sure a lot more interest than anyone at the VA ever showed.

"Sounds like a pretty solid case to me," John said, reaching for a legal pad and a pair of pens. "Let's outline exactly what we want done."

Yep, I thought, he *is* a note taker. Order and organization; I liked that. I had my list already composed mentally, so together we sipped coffee — yes, *this* office provided hospitality — and drew it up.

CHARLES LEWIS   CASE NUMBER XYZ-000-000

TO BE ACCOMPLISHED BY VA

1. Establish service connection for Crohn's Disease.

2. Establish service connection date as January 1981. Veterans Administration failed to notify vet-

eran of his rights to appeal, and did not honor his request to be evaluated for Crohn's.

3. Reimburse all medical expenses veteran paid out of pocket. Payment is owed due to VA's neglect of veteran's medical problems contracted while on tour of duty.

4. Re-rate disability at 100%. Veteran is unemployable because of advanced and serious status of Crohn's disease. (Note: It is unlikely that the disease would have progressed to this disabling status if the VA had properly treated the condition at its onset.)

5. Formally evaluate for Post Traumatic Stress Disorder (PTSD). Veteran has been diagnosed with PTSD but the VA failed to follow up by entering the condition on medical records, and such is not reflected on his disability rating.

After we completed the handwritten draft and John tapped out a formatted document on his word processor, we reviewed it item by item. "It's hard to believe the VA has ignored you for so long," he said, "but your requests are specific and the details give teeth to them. The VA will give you static about the time that's elapsed since your original physical in 1981, but with the documentation you have in your own possession, we can clear that hurdle."

John's strategy: attack one issue at a time. "We'll combine the evaluation for Crohn's disease and PTSD into one physical. Once we establish the service connections, then we go for retroactive benefits. After those are accomplished, we address each other issue in turn."

"Yeah," I agreed. "It's not a good idea to overwhelm them with a bunch of requests at once because it only slows them up. The VA has a big problem doing more than one thing at a time, like walking and chewing gum."

Then I told John my family was in deep trouble financially, and on welfare, and I would really appreciate getting this going and completed in the fastest mode possible. "I'm just not in any mood to have the VA continue to procrastinate on this for another year or six," I said, "because if they do, they'll only have to incur one more expense on my behalf. That will be when they bury me, because they are essentially administering euthanasia."

Then I signed a Power of Attorney allowing the DAV to represent me, and to have access to my files.

As I arranged and tidied my papers, John asked me about the incident up at the VA office that morning.

"Gee, does the grapevine grow up the walls here or what?" I asked, surprised that he'd heard. As far as I knew, John had been here all the time.

Anyway, since he asked, I gave him the color commentary. While I did, John kept shaking his head, looking disgusted. I couldn't tell whether it was with the VA, or with my behavior.

Discussing the day as we drove home, Tina and I concluded that I should not have tried to take on the VA alone, but should have gotten a service rep from the very start.

"Don't work with the VA any more by yourself, Chuck. It's clear you can no longer deal with them in a rational manner."

"I could deal with the VA in a very rational manner if they would take my case seriously and do the job they were employed to do," I shot back. "Hell, the place is a goddamned revolving door ... line 'em up in the morning, put hash marks on the wall for every one you tell you don't know anything, and send glowing reports to Washington about how many vets you're, quote, serving."

"Okay, they are not an efficient machine. But regardless of how screwed up the bureaucracy is, you don't do yourself any good by firing on their ass. Chuck, I'm totally embarrassed by your conduct. Don't ask me to go to the VA with you again because I won't."

Now if that isn't a hell of a note! I am a disabled vet trying to get what the law says I have coming to me. Since when is a man supposed to allow someone to put him and his family in the dump and keep him there?

"Well, Hon, short of re-enlisting in the service I can see no way out of our present circumstances. Re-enlisting is out of the question, for obvious reasons."

Tina sort of smirked, then diverted the conversation to Andrea. *Now what in the name of the world does she have up her sleeve this time?*

As soon we arrived home I went straight to our neighbor's to use his phone. (That was a necessity we could not afford.) I called Congressman Elliott in Washington — surprise! he was in his office — and he listened to the tale of my morning.

"I really needed all the help you came through with, Sir, and I can never thank you enough for that," I told him. "I turned my case over to John at the DAV. I am sure his influence will be necessary, and that he has the personality and clout to get the VA off their sorry asses and get to work on my case."

"I think John is your man," Elliott said. "I'll get in touch, do what I can to help him along."

"Right now my life has about completely fallen apart and at this point I'm getting desperate. I don't know how much longer I can deal with this bucket of muck."

I ended up getting an appointment with Elliott's Seattle aide for the following Monday.

Maybe this time, I thought.

16

When I got back to our apartment, Tina was at the table, surrounded by an array of Technicolor pamphlets. I told her about my conversation with Congressman Elliott, then asked, "What've you got there?"

"Brochures."

"From . . . ?"

"The Coast Guard."

"What's that all about?"

"Enlisting. Like you said."

"You mean when we were watching that jazzy commercial in December? Hell, Babe, I wasn't *serious*!"

"I'm in the checking-it-out stage right now. But when it's decision-making time, it's my decision, not yours."

I joined her at the table and looked over the papers with their slick-em sales pitch. All the services use it, telling about all the neat-o, life-enriching, personally expanding, character-building, enabling, empowering experiences one is "allowed" by choosing this branch of the military. It failed to mention all the outrages you have to deal with in order to take advantage of the neat-o things.

Andrea arrived home from school, and while I fixed supper I listened to her bubbly reports of her day at the education institute. How I adored her childlike enthusiasm!

Meanwhile, Tina went to the neighbor's to call the Coast Guard recruiter and set up an appointment for Friday.

What mixed-up feelings churned around inside me! On one hand I was so proud of this woman who would go to such an extreme to keep her family together, to back up her husband who, despite his efforts, was unable to meet his obligations to his family. God, I was so proud of her! I thought about how most women would trash their husbands for not being able to take care of them. And, well ... Tina had done her share of that, too, for a fact.

I feel an ulterior motive slithering around me. Over the past five years Tina's behavior has consisted of one shitball scene after another. Oh, fergodsake blow it off, Lewis. Don't worry about stuff unless it happens. *Right, Voice On My Shoulder. Maybe this time Tina is truly doing something for her family.*

Tina's appointment with the recruiter was in two days, and we used the time to discuss the things she would have to deal with if she were to join the Coast Guard. Her age — 29 — and having to compete with younger, fitter kids, and her having to take orders from people younger than herself. The grunge details she would be expected to do (which gave me cause for concern; she *never* lowered herself to clean a toilet or scrub a wall for *us*).

I soothed, "It isn't going to be easy on you. But you have experience, maturity, and knowledge of real life going in your favor. I also pledge my unconditional support and all the experience in my background to help you along."

Tina had decreed that she'd never again go to the VA with me, but that didn't mean she didn't want *me* going with *her* to her interview with the recruiter. So on Friday we set out for Seattle and reported to the United States Coast Guard.

To the recruiter's apparent surprise, Tina told him firmly that she wanted to enlist right then and there. She had with her all the documents she would need for enlistment. "Of course I don't expect to be able to get sworn in today, but I'm prepared to start the paperwork," she explained.

While Tina filled out papers I grabbed a cup of coffee and looked over the recruiting propaganda "attractively arranged" on the reception room rack. A man whose nameplate said he was the in-house commander sauntered over.

"You'll look quite different with your long hair cut off and your beard shaved," he said in a tone that tried to be joshing-friendly.

"Whoa, man. My wife is the one joining. I already gave this country over thirteen years of my life. While I was on active duty the United States Government was my best friend, but now that I am out it has become my worst enemy. I am what some people refer to as a Disabled Veteran who can't get any help. I couldn't pass your entrance physical if someone else took it for me."

The commander sat down and had coffee with me as he asked about my military career. Then he offered, "We're pretty surprised at the number of people getting out of the regular branches of the service and joining the Coast Guard."

"A lot of them get turned loose into society and then find they prefer the military community," I told him, in case he didn't know why people re-enlisted. "And too many vets, especially 'Nam vets, especially those with any disabilities, are finding it really hard to get decent jobs," I said.

The commander's eyes swept me up and down. "My friends who are heads of business firms tell me that a lot of people show up for interviews looking so anti-authority and anti-society that they'd close down before they'd hire a protester-type. If people put on a professional appearance they'd be a whole lot more employable."

I bet this guy is talking about ME. He wants me to get a haircut, trim my beard, and wear a tie. Well, that's just *his* opinion.

When Tina reappeared, she had appointments for a Monday afternoon entrance exam and a Tuesday morning physical.

With high hopes we headed out to my Monday morning meeting with Congressman Elliot's aide and Tina's exams that afternoon. I hadn't felt too red-hot the whole night before, so Tina got to be the one to navigate Seattle's maze of one-way streets. But true to her vow not to accompany me to any more such meetings, she stayed in the car, grabbing some exam-cram time (and nervously chain-smoking).

I think the aide was a practicum student. A second-quarter-senior political science major, no doubt, getting ten hours of credit and a tiny stipend that couldn't possibly have covered the tab for his brand-new Young Yuppie Career Wear three-piece suit.

I introduced myself, then thanked the lad for the outstanding sleuthwork the congressman had done on my behalf.

"The congressman has, like, done just about all he can do at this point," smiled The Suit. "With his help as your launch, you are now, y'know, free to pursue your case as you see appropriate."

That's politalk for 'I'm dumped.' Congressman Elliott knocked himself out being helpful; this young yup is in a totally different universe. Yeah, Lewis, all youngsters in the bureauforce are like that, haven't you noticed? *Yep, they're impotents on a power trip. I think they somehow feel they're getting even with their parents. All people over 35 are their parents.*

I told The Suit what happened at the VA office the prior week, but he appeared unmoved.

"Well, an individual congressman has, like, y'know, limited power, and Mr. Elliott can not, y'know, intervene any further. However," the Powerkid smiled again, "you can, like, rest assured that you are not the only one with, y'know, this type of problem. Sometimes it just takes time to, like, get things, y'know, straightened out."

"*TIME*, you say? My claim has been going on a few days over six goddamned years!"

A United States Congressman claiming no authority to help a constituent having a problem with an agency of the United States Government? What kind of a run-around is this ten-credit little God-impostor spinning me here?

I left the congressman's office feeling like a rat in a cage. No exit, no destination. Just running and running on a wheel that goes nowhere.

On the way to the testing center I tried to calm Tina's nervousness. I reminded her how well she had done on the same test to get in the Army. "Besides, Hon, with the experience and education you've gained, you can handle that idiot-factor test with one hand and no sweat."

As Tina jumped through her hoops it was my turn to sit in the car, smoking and mulling. My body signaled the oncoming of another flare-up — tenderness in the abdomen, cramps coming more often and more fiercely. Tomorrow I will see Dr. Fien. Right now, while Tina prepares to join the Coast Guard, is no time to find myself laid out in bed.

When Tina returned, she saw that I was in distress. She took the wheel and drove straight to Dr. Fien's. *Tina's changing back into the woman I fell in love with. She didn't say a word about herself; her first concern was for me.*

We hit Dr. Fien between patients. I didn't even have to choose which shop-worn magazine not to read while I waited; he took me right in. He examined me, prescribed another batch of medication, and set another appointment for the following week.

"This is four different medications now, Doctor, I'm having major difficulty with that. I'm not one for even popping an aspirin for a headache."

"Take them," he ordered.

Tina drove us home. I almost made it into the house ... almost. Damn, this is so humiliating. And added to the humiliation is fear, the fear that Tina will grow so disgusted with a husband who craps his pants that one day she'll slip out into the night and dissolve from my life.

Suddenly very weak and very, very ill (I felt like a molded Jell-O and moved with about the same agility), I woggled myself into bed. Tina threw my clothes in the wash, then came in and sat on the edge of the bed.

"Since we're old soldiers and all, let's talk about a battle plan to attack the VA," she said.

"VA? There is no VA. It isn't real, none of this is real. The VA says I do not have Crohn's, I am not ill, and I am not disabled. If this devil's pain inside me is not real, then I am not real ... so you, my dear, are a single woman."

"Well, it's real enough that I have come to understand and accept that you might never get any long-time work. That's why I made the decision to join the Coast Guard. With your disability compensation plus my income, we can make it. Or at least be better off than we are now. We'd pay lower rent for government housing and utilities, and as a dependent, you would be able to get medical treatment when you need it."

And she still hasn't talked about herself. My old girlfriend is back and these dampened eyes are not from the pain in my innards.

The next morning Tina went to Seattle for her physical and to take the final steps to enlisting.

In no shape to go anywhere, I stayed home to grapple with my VA dilemma. I wandered to our next door neighbor's and bounced the scenario around with her. "Is there a source of assistance outside the governmental system that might be willing to take on the VA?" I wondered aloud.

"Like a lawyer, for example?" she suggested.

Using her phone (*Remember to scrape up some cash and pay a portion of her phone bill before you move, Lewis!*), I wrote names, numbers, and specialties of a score or so of Seattle area lawyers listed in the yellow pages and began making calls. What I got was: stonewalled. As soon as I said, "VA" the discussion was over.

Finally, I got to the last lawyer on my list. This one did not hang up when I said *VA*.

"You aren't going to find anyone to represent you," the attorney told me, "because there is still a law on the books that says a veteran can pay an attorney only ten dollars for counsel in matters pertaining to his military service."

Still on the books?" I asked, too stunned to fume. "As in it's been there a long time? Since when?"

"Since the law was passed during the Civil War era."

"Wait a damn minute," I said. "Either my hearing loss is greater than the VA admits or I'm as crazy as the VA shrink says I am. Will you run that by me again?" He did, and I was neither deaf nor crazy.

"Well, the law does make sense in the respect that it keeps a veteran from being ripped off by an unscrupulous attorney," I said, beginning to recover enough to start fuming. "But no change in fee structure for A HUNDRED AND FORTY YEARS?!"

"Well, it's legal to be *represented* by counsel," he said, sounding defensive. "You just can't pay more than ten dollars."

So why do we keep hearing about all these charity cases lawyers take on? The scum who push drugs on street corners, the scam artists and cop-killers whom attorneys defend for a song, then sanctimoniously call it public service? I didn't say it aloud, I was listening to Voice On My Shoulder; so the legal-eagle must have taken my silence to mean I concurred with this B.S. nonsense, and he inhaled and plunged onward.

"The Veterans Administration is protected by law from being taken to Federal court," the lawyer explained. "The VA cannot be sued."

"So you're saying veterans are denied the very constitutional rights they fought wars to defend? Amazing!"

I had followed the news of riots in the Louisiana and Atlanta Federal prisons, where illegal immigrants who were designated as criminals were about to be deported to Cuba. Their response was: Riot. They caused millions of dollars of damage and the deaths of several people. No action was taken against them until the Federal court heard their case. These people were criminals, and not even citizens — and I doubt any of them had even ten dollars to purchase counsel — yet they have more constitutional rights to American courts of law than a veteran who honorably served his country. What happened to the First Amendment and the right to petition the government for redress of grievances? Is this a constitutional right given up when one serves our country? I am sure glad I have been enlightened to this little tidbit that gives me second or third class citizenship of the country I served.

Tina returned home to report her physical went great, and she expected to get enlisted within a week or two.

In turn I reported spending the afternoon with a phone in my ear, relating what I found out from the one lawyer who'd talk with me about it.

"I can't believe all this crap!" she exclaimed, and she began railing about all the things I had railed about. Her anger fed mine, and we got very full.

In the morning I called John at the DAV. "I'm going to continue to bug you about pushing my case," I told him. "And be warned: I am not going to quit and let them win."

Tina reported to Cape May, New Jersey for boot camp and Andrea and I stayed in Kent. "No use packing up and trekking across the continent for that short a time, because I *shall* be stationed on the West Coast," she assured me.

We heard little from her. "Too busy to write," she wrote.

Too busy to send our allotment, too? We hadn't gotten a cent. Later, I found that the Coast Guard withholds all but a coffee-and-newspaper amount of allowance until recruits graduate from training. The Coast Guard had failed to mention this "policy," and when Tina failed to send the expected rent money, Andrea and I came *this close* to being evicted. She said many of her classmates' dependents were left as high, dry, and broke as we were. When I knew why Tina had sent me no money, I felt embarrassed, guilty, and foolish for getting angry and suspicious.

While Tina was gone and during the hours Andrea was at school, I became practically a fixture at the library. In my investigation I discovered that the U.S. Supreme Court had heard arguments on the issue of claims and appeals. In one class action suit, the Court ruled that veterans do not need to go to Federal court, that the VA has enough of its own checks and balances.

Now what kind of fucking decision was that! All the so-called checks and balances are within the system — from one VA official to another, all within the same fiefdom, one self-appointed noble to another. This atrocity of a law allows for no "disinterested third party," no right of appeal clear to the Supreme Court

— the very keystone of the First Amendment and of our legal system. For everyone except veterans.

Sure, the VA can retort that *all* the veterans' service organizations — VFW, American Legion, AmVets, DAV, and so on — do indeed represent veterans in their claims against the VA. But not Vietnam vets. It's no secret that those organizations have an historical record for ignoring them. Vietnam was, after all, an undeclared war, and engaging in it and escalating it was wrong. So the organizations apparently use that as the excuse to rule that the 'Nam vet isn't a veteran in the true sense of the word. They are accepted for membership purposes — pronounced *We take your money* — but not until the mid-nineteen nineties would they really be accepted as brother veterans.

Life, as the comedians say, is full of little ironies. The VA says the disabilities I incurred in combat are not service related; and the Veterans of Foreign Wars says don't sweat the point, because I'm not a veteran anyway.

The date of Tina's graduation from boot camp happened to coincide with a special promotion co-sponsored by an airline and a supermarket chain. Buy a hundred dollars worth of groceries and you could buy a one-way ticket to anywhere in the U.S. for fifty bucks. I had everyone I knew saving receipts for me and I bought two tickets to New York City. Andrea and I would stay with Tina's parents, and I would drive Pop's car to Cape May, three hours away.

Andrea and I arrived a week before graduation so that I could go to the Cape and spend the weekend with my wife. It was the only off-post pass she was allowed the whole basic training period.

The way I was anticipating a romantic and sexy reunion made me feel like a giddy college kid. But it didn't turn out that way. Tina seemed . . . aloof . . . no, probably stressed and tired. We checked into our motel and went to dinner. We took in a movie, then met some of her cohorts and went out with them for drinks.

Tina's hoped for assignment to the West Coast didn't turn out, either. She would be stationed at Sandy Hook, New Jersey. We decided that after graduation, while on our way back to New

York, I would contact the housing officer in Sandy Hook and apply for quarters for the three of us.

I called Mrs. Thomas, the warrant officer in charge of housing. She advised that before she could assign the family a quarters, Tina would have to sign into the post first. So it was decided: We would all go to Sandy Hook, get our quarters assignment, fly to Seattle, pack, then drive back to New Jersey.

After the graduation exercises we picked up Tina's things and hit the road. She had only ten days of leave before having to report to duty. In that time we had to make a coast-to-coast round trip and close up a household in between. I called home to ask my mom to conjure up three more of those fifty dollar plane tickets.

Sandy Hook is a peninsula that is part of Gateway National Recreation Area. Except for the Coast Guard station, the area is operated by the National Park Service. Beauty all around! Space. A waterfront. People pay small fortunes to live in the vicinity — and here we were, *assigned* to be there, and at the low-rent rate to boot. Most important to me, it is quiet, isolated from the sardine-can chaos that is the typical East Coast lifestyle.

While Tina reported to station headquarters, Andrea twirled round and round, admiring the panorama and chattering excitedly about living here. She was describing so many things she would do she practically had my ears smokin'.

While I listened to Andrea's effervescence, I notice the POW/MIA flag flying over the station. Public display of that flag commemorates those still unaccounted for and also reminds America of the tragedies of the Vietnam War. As I found out later, all New Jersey state agencies must fly the POW/MIA flag along with the Stars and Stripes. Coast Guard Station Sandy Hook, being a federal installation, was not required to fly the flag but it did so.

As I also found out later, a lot of ex-POWs live in that area and they visit the Hook, proud of what that flag represents. Though it started out commemorating the prisoners of war and those missing in action in Vietnam, it now symbolizes all POWs and MIAs of all our wars.

It was gratifying to see that flag flying at the station. It was gratifying, too, that Andrea saw it and mentioned it. It made a wonderful teaching opportunity.

When Tina was officially checked in, the three of us went to meet Mrs. Thomas. We signed on the line and suddenly we had a new home. We went to look at it. It was an upstairs apartment and it had only one bathroom.

"Oh, dear, this isn't going to work," I said, dismayed. Then I explained my medical problem, telling her, "During a Crohn's attack I can't deal with the stairs."

"This is the last empty apartment on the base," she said kindly. "You really need a town house, but if you don't accept this apartment I'm afraid your only choices would be either to live in town at your own expense, or your dependents," Mrs. Thomas addressed Tina, "would have to stay in Seattle until there's a town house available on base."

Tina and I looked at each other. What to do?

"However, because your medical problem is a special-circumstance situation, Mr. Lewis, I can assure you that you folks will get the next available unit if you want to accept this one until then. You'd sort of be in a holding pattern."

We accepted the apartment with that understanding.

Then it was off to New York. Tina's family turned out, the whole clan of them, congratulating her on her enlistment-graduation-station assignment, telling Andrea My, How You've Grown, and having a nice reunion in general. Tina had not seen them for two years.

They still had no idea of what we had been going through. Every time Tina phoned or wrote she painted them a pretty picture of our lives. Her deception bothered me, but on the other hand, she had spared them the worry.

The next morning we flew to Seattle. We arrived exhausted. Rather than driving back to our hovel, we spent the night with Mom and Dad.

The following morning I let Tina and Andrea sleep in while I went to our apartment. With Tina's allotment allowance finally in hand, I paid up the back rent and cheerfully informed the landlady we were getting out of her ragbag firetrap. I paid all our bills, arranged to rent a U-Haul, and arranged for the shipping of everything else we couldn't fit in the trailer.

The next three days whooshed by in a blur of sorting and packing, and of good-byes to the few people who really counted. Like Ted. He came over to help, and we couldn't have gotten the apartment packed and cleaned in the allotted time without him.

"After all, we were practically betrothed," Ted said as he loaded up another box of trash to carry down to the dumpster. "Being partners in a business is a serious as marriage, you know."

"I'm sorry it didn't work out; that's my biggest regret," I said. "We proved one thing, though. We proved that people who really need business loans can't get them. Banks lend money who people who already have assets equal to the amount they want to borrow."

"Well, look at it this way," Ted said cheerfully. "If we had managed to start the business, we'd be dissolving a partnership right now, because you're moving."

"Ted, if we'd'a gotten that business opened up, I wouldn't *need* to be moving."

We set out cross-continent. It was a noteworthy journey because for once (for the first time in the history of mankind, perhaps) Murphy's Law did not kick in. (You know Murphy's Law: "Everything takes longer than you thought; if anything can go wrong, it will.") Seattle to Sandy Hook, New Jersey in four days.

PART TWO

17

We arrived in Sandy Hook on a Wednesday in April of 1987. Since Tina didn't have to check in until Friday, we unhitched the U-Haul, parked it in front of our new apartment, and went up to New York City to see Tina's mom and pop. I wanted to stay, unpack, and get rooted; besides, we had seen the old folks less than two weeks before. But Tina insisted, so we went — with my grave misgivings, for I feared Tina was experiencing the onset of mama-dependency.

We arrived back at The Hook on Friday. A whole weekend to relax and settle in before Tina's first shift on Monday! Nevertheless, she got her papers together and headed to headquarters to formally report for duty. I started unloading the trailer and taking things upstairs to the apartment. Andrea did what six-year-olds normally do: she went to the playground to discover what was available to climb and swing on.

Soon Tina returned with a shocker. She had to report for work right away. The station brass gave her no time to settle in, nor did they give us any Welcome Wagon-type information about the place, no lists of local stores and services ... nothing. She would be on duty straight through to Monday morning.

What kind of leadership do they have at this place? Of my many moves to many military bases, this was the first time a service person with a family was not given a day or two to get settled and oriented. *Hey, don't go blaming "the leadership" one hundred percent. You could have stayed here to get your stuff together, you know, instead of running to Mommie and Poppy*

Not one person stopped, came by, called, visited, or asked if we needed help, directions, advice, or a hand. It was as if no one was interested in Tina the person, but only in Tina the new recruit and the extra pair of hands. The persona of a station is established by its leadership. I had experienced this type of leadership in the Army, and units under such command normally had discipline problems and low morale.

We wasted a fair amount of time doing it, but Andrea and I, on our own, found the best supermarket and located the U-Haul drop station. Then we went exploring our front yard — the beach.

We had an awesome view of the bay; if I wanted to, I could cast my fishing line from my bedroom window. Andrea and I sat on the sea wall and watched the water, mesmerized. This incredible place was to be our home for at least the next few years.

Tina returned home from her shift just after nine o'clock Monday morning. She didn't have to report back until Wednesday morning. Two on, two off: This was to be her rotating duty schedule, with alternate weekends free.

Tina's first month in the Coast Guard whizzed by. Everthing went unbelievably well. The only problem I saw was that people were generally bored during their off-duty time, and that created a marginally bad drinking problem. Thank goodness Tina had her family to occupy her energies and her obligations, plus the several years of maturity and life experience she had over the majority of enlisted personnel here. By virtue of her family status, partying and carousing would hold no lure for her. I thought.

I called the Veterans Administration Regional Office in Newark, asking them to get my records from the Seattle VARO. Just to double-jump-start the process, I also called Seattle and asked them to send my files to Newark.

I also requested the Newark Disabled American Veterans chapter to procure my records from their Seattle office. Then I called John at the DAV in Seattle and asked him to see that my records get transferred quickly and properly to New Jersey.

Having done that kind of cross-requesting, I sat back, anticipating getting all my records transferred.

With Tina working, I became househusband and Andrea's primary caretaker. Prior to our departure from Kent, Andrea had "graduated" from kindergarten early. "Now I'm a Big Girl," Andrea said proudly, and I agreed. Just a month away from turning six, she was brighter and more perceptive than other children her age. Accordingly, I believed she would learn more and develop greater maturity and responsibility at my side than she would in a classroom, so I chose not to enroll her in preschool here. She became my right-hand helper and buddy. She helped me with the shopping and became my junior homemaker. I bought her a fishing pole. We packed bags of muchies and juice and spent afternoons exploring, adventuring, and joking about living off the bounty of the sea.

Andrea soaked up a stunning storehouse of knowledge and understanding. She learned to read a tide table, and began to grasp the fundamental physics and mathematics of tides. She learned about tidepools and estuaries, about ecologies and life forms and patterns of succession from the depths of the sea to points inland, and began to to read cloudbanks and wind patterns. In the fall she'd have to give up all this learning time to start first grade, and to See Dick Run.

Tina's job title was Boat Engineer. She was the only female engine mechanic on the station, a point of pride for us both. However, she was under a time deadline to make a bunch of qualifications to keep her rating and advance. Rather than hitting the manuals and boning up, though, she spent many of her off-duty days in New York. Now I was okay with her making up some lost time with her family, but we still needed a lot of household stuff, and every trip to New York cost at least a hundred dollars.

It also cost a lot in domestic tranquility. I simply was not physically up to making the frequent trips, and I dared not participate in family outings taking us far from amenities as they did. Even after all these years, I could not make these people understand the nature of my illness — hell, I couldn't convince them I was ill at all; they continued preferring the idea that I'm just another wacked-out vet, using it as an excuse to be anti-social.

I couldn't understand why everyone wanted to make such an issue of my not "Familying." (It was such a sacred concept they used it as a verb). None of them liked me, nor I them. I am convinced they made it an issue solely and only because it gave them something to bitch about.

Soon Tina added another diversion, and it met what I cynically called her top requirements. (A) It kept her from having to be at home; (B) It allowed her to drop lots of money. All of a sudden she began going into town with the guys on her shift, spending her days off at a local pub. She came home from work, got herself decked out — make-up, hairdo, doll-baby clothes (I do not know when she bought those risque outfits, nor where, nor with what) — and off she went until the small morning hours.

Now, I didn't have a big problem with her going out and schmoozing with her duty section after a long shift of work. But damn it all, she seldom went out with *me* ... and when she did, she didn't bother with a comb or lipstick or even fresh jeans. I was deeply hurt; but I figured this was just a phase and she'd pass through it.

By the first of May, nearly two months after contacting all the offices and departments of the VA, the Newark office answered my question: My records had not arrived from Seattle. Same story at DAV: The guy who "was going to" assign a caseworker to me still had not done a thing.

God, Lewis, if they can't handle a kindergarten-level task like putting a folder in an envelope and mailing it, what makes you think they can handle an appeal?

After I made a few pointed remarks to the powers that be, the Newark office assigned me a case worker —*another new guy. Sigh* — named Harry.

"Can't understand the ineptitude," Harry said. "It shouldn't take more than one request and no more than a week or so to get a file transferred. At any rate I'll hound Seattle to get those records out, and I'll start expediting your claim as soon as I have the papers."

Tina devised a weekly schedule: two duty tours and one two-day, off-duty party with the guys at work, plus a couple of trips to New York per month. Her Me-First pursuits of pleasure were bleeding us financially.

And now she cooked up yet another outlet for her cash. She had to have her own TV and her own stereo in her duty room. And tools: The government issue tools in the shop weren't good enough, or not specialized enough, so she went out and bought her own. We have no bed, and car maintenance is long overdue, but by cracky, *her* TV is better than the station-issue one in her section's lounge.

She went through money so quickly I couldn't even keep up with our recordkeeping. One day our bank account had a reasonable balance and the next day it was gone. Tina said she made money and she deserved things.

And gone. She was always gone. One day Andrea asked me, "Will Mommy do something with us on her day off? Or will she go out with the guys?"

"I don't know, Honey."

It seemed a perfect opening for having things out with Tina. Just after nine the next morning she came in from her duty shift. She went straight to the closet and started pushing hangers around, looking for an outfit.

"Andrea was hoping for some Mommy-daughter time today," I said carefully, dipping a toe in the water.

Silence.

"She misses her mother, Tina. And that's to your credit."

"If you were doing your part to keep her entertained, she wouldn't have time to miss her mommy."

She's really dipping low for excuses, but this one is too preposterous to dignify. "Tina, I acknowledge your role as the breadwinner here," I said, not bothering to add that she hadn't yet given one crumb of her bread to the household. "And that gives you a lot of entitlements. But a child needs her mother."

"Well, you and Andrea will have to accept that *I* need some *space* for a while."

"I understand your need for space, Tina. But stepping out on your spouse? Ignoring your six-year-old? Spending days at a time in the pub? Is that the kind of space you need?"

"Oh, shut up, Chuck! I see you're calling on your cherished 'stress syndrome' again as an excuse to overreact. Nothing is going on with me and my crew."

Tina put on a dress which I hope to hell she got for half price because it only half covered her, and stalked out the door. Andrea got out one of those little touch-and-fuzzy books from her babyhood and she curled up very small in a corner and sucked her thumb and quietly wept.

Tina's dad called that morning. "Is Tina there? Can I talk to my baby?"

"As a matter of fact, she isn't, Pop. She's at the pub with all the single young horny guys on her shift crew. Andrea is crying for her mommy because Mommy is always either at work or at a party, and your granddaughter feels rejected. Help me out here, Pop — how does a man get his wife to come to her senses?"

"You're disgusting, Chuck. You're crazy, even thinking such things."

Three major occupations filled my time. Andrea. The VA. Job hunting.

Trying to find a job was a waste of time, for all the same old reasons.

Not working really got to me. Why couldn't I have simply been killed like my buddies? Maybe Tina's attitude toward me was justified, after all. *Stand apart and look at yourself, Lewis: Would you want to have yourself around?*

How could one be such a good soldier and such a loser in civilian life?

It isn't just the startle-and-react to every loud and sudden sound. It's the constant annoyance with . . . everything. The insincerity, fluffiness, and incompetence of the business world. The ineptness and lack of empathy and all the excuse making. And my wife running around on me.

Maybe Tina is right; I guess the PTSD is stalking me again; and it is a more serious and demoralizing condition than even the never-been-in-combat shrinks and sociologists think it is.

18

May melted into June and nothing changed, except that Andrea grew in wisdom and stature and self-reliance, and in the ability to divine what was going on with adults, even the ones who ignored her.

The headquarters building housed the station post office. People converged there, milling around, visiting. Who you expecting to hear from? Who *did* you hear from? Let's see if you and I got the same junk mail.

On this balmy day near June's end my friend Tim and I showed up before mail call to visit, as we did, more and more frequently. Tim was a line officer in Tina's crew and I told him a little about Nam and the VA, but never, ever did I share any details or information about the pain Tina was putting me through.

"I'm still looking for a letter from the VA," I told him, extracting the mail from my box.

"The one you've been expecting for two months?"

"Well, today's the day! Look!" I said, waving the envelope with the Seattle Veterans Administration Regional Office return address.

Eagerly, I tore open the envelope and withdrew the letter and held it so Tim could read it with me, share the good news as soon as I got it.

> Dear Mr. Lewis:
>
> Since you did not report for your scheduled examination, we have no choice but to deny your claim for service connection for Post Traumatic Stress Disorder and Crohn's Disease.
>
> We cannot take further action unless you inform us of your willingness to report for an

examination by signing the statement below and returning this letter to us at the address shown above. We will then re-schedule your examination and reconsider your claim when the examination is completed.

IMPORTANT: Please show your full name and VA file number on all correspondence or evidence submitted.

If you believe our decision is incorrect, please see the Notice of Procedural and Appellate Rights printed on the back of this letter.

Sincerely yours,

V. A.

cc: D. A. V.

Tim flashed me a puzzled look and watched me go ballistic.

"I CAN NOT BELIEVE THIS PIECE OF BUTT WIPE!" I bellowed. "Fuck this letter and the clerk who typed it and fuck the whole damn lazy cheap incompetent frigging V fucking A!"

Tim had stepped away and his eyes fixed on something fascinating on the wall behind me, but everyone else stopped still in their tracks and stared. I stomped through the building and onto the porch and through the crowd outside, raging as I went.

"Three months since we moved to New Jersey, Seaman," I yelled, addressing the first fellow who happened to be on my pathway. "I sent *TWO REQUESTS* through every channel the VA ever heard of, asking Seattle to get my files transferred — " and I turned to Christy, one of Tina's friends and just about the only woman Tina never made snippy comments about, "— and I get this, Christy —" I waved the letter in the startled woman's face "— as if I never moved or anything has happened. Even though they KNEW I moved they still set up an appointment knowing I could not be there."

I hooked my arm through the arm of the next fellow along the way. "Do you see what the VA did?" I demanded. Wide-eyed, he shook his head. "I'll tell what the VA did. They made an appointment for me to be in a place I moved from three months ago and told them I moved. They cleverly and deliberately created documentation they could use to show I failed to cooperate with their agency. My records and files should have been in Newark two months before this letter —" I waved it in his face "— was even generated."

I turned to the next onlooker unfortunate enough to be next to me. "Look at this asinine laugh line," I said, pointing to the letter's first sentence and reading it loudly for all to hear. '*Since you did not report for your scheduled examination* —" What 'schedule'? I did not ever receive one word, one letter, postcard, phone call, carrier pigeon, or ham radio relay saying I had any schedule for any meeting, appointment, examination, or pop quiz at the esteemed United States Veterans Administration. So why is it," I looked the onlooker in the eye, "that the VA can send a letter to my correct address informing me that I didn't *keep* their freaking appointment, when they couldn't find me to inform me I *had* an appointment to begin with?"

The fellow shook loose from my grasp and retreated into the crowd without answering. So I collared the next person in reach.

"You work for the glorious Federal Bureau of Veterans Administration?" I asked, holding my mail in one hand and a wad of his shirt in the other.

The guy clicked his heels. "No, SIR!"

I let go of the man's shirt — "Sorry about the wrinkles," I mumbled — and strode through the crowd which parted before me like the Red Sea as I bee-lined for the shop where Tina was working.

I handed Tina the letter and explained it to her crewmates as she read. She looked astonished but retained her composure.

"Did you notice this little epistle doesn't have a signature?" I asked, refusing to be calmed by her collectedness. "The sorry bastard who wrote it doesn't even the intestinal fortitude to sign his or her own name."

"I see that a courtesy copy of the letter was supposedly sent to the DAV," Tina observed, pointing to the *CC* at the bottom.

"So where the hell *is* this jerk DAV assistant-slash advocate-slash representative?" I fumed. "He was the first person I informed about our change of address, and he's the one who was supposed to inform everyone else and get all my records sent here. And he didn't notice all this mail was being sent to an extinct address? This is the representative I am supposed to trust to handle my case?"

"What are you going to do next?" Tina asked, still calm.

"I'm going home and run up the phone bill, and get to the bottom of it all. I have questions I want answered, and I want my answers now." I consulted my watch. "Almost five o'clock here; that's still prime-time working hours on the west coast — in case they work on the west coast, which I doubt."

As I departed station headquarters the flag was being retired for the day. Proper protocol for honoring the retiring of the colors is to stop all activity and stand at attention until the flag is lowered. This time, though, I ignored all that and burst right through the center of the ceremony.

The petty officer in charge didn't like that all. He stopped me and tried to make an issue.

"Mr. Petty, I was actively serving that tricolored piece of cloth when you were still being potty trained. I have served that symbol in war and in peace, and if anyone has a right to take it to issue, I am the one. I can not respect what does not respect me."

In unison the color guardsmen moved forward a step as if to forcibly remove me, but I held up a hand and they stopped.

"That piece of cloth represents a government I served faithfully for over thirteen years, and when I need something in return all its representatives can do is blow me off." I met the Coast Guardsmen eye for eye. "Well fuck them and the flag they claim to represent. I am fed up with the government representatives' horse-shit, jaw-flapping excuses."

Over the assemblage's audible gasp I said, "If anyone ever had the right to degrade our country's symbol, I have, because I have fought, been wounded, and am permanently and incurably disabled for the right to do so. I no longer have to live up to any oath to protect the flag or any goddamned thing else, especially a Constitution that denies me my rights to due process after I have faithfully served it."

I swept my eyes over the group of fifteen or so Coasties participating in the Retiring of the Colors ceremony. "I give you an old American blessing which I just made up," I said, and I raised an open palm above them as if I were a priest. "May you never be called upon to fight for your country, but if you are, may you never be hurt, wounded, maimed, or disabled, for your country will find a loophole to deny you any compensation."

Then I faced the petty officer and said, "If you don't like it you can take a swing at me right here and now, but if you do, you'll have this fucking flag draped over your fucking casket."

I turned to leave, fully expecting to get shot in the back or at least jumped. Let them, I thought. I was adrenalized enough to take them all on.

Nobody jumped. Nobody booed, gestured, or catcalled. In silence, they parted and let me pass.

Christy awaited me at the apartment doorway. Andrea held Christy's right hand and her five-year-old Betsy held the other, and each little girl held a Fudgesickle in her free hand.

"Hi, Chuck. How 'bout if Andrea comes to play with Betsy? She can stay for dinner and some playground time if that's okay with you." Christy's eyes met mine. "Take some private time," she whispered.

I threw Andrea a kiss and I squeezed Christy's shoulder.

You worry too much about nobody understanding, Lewis. Some people do, you know.

I climbed the steps to the apartment and jumped right on the phone and started my calls.

The first jerk I called was my so-called representative at the DAV in Seattle. The best this sorry piece of future worm food could do was make ten thousand excuses for his foul-up.

"You can rest assured I will personally take care of the situation and get everything straightened out," he said, all formal-pleasant, arm's length business.

That, I recognized by now, is Standard Dismissal #1 ... and the pleasanter the voice, the worse the snafu it's covering up.

"If you had done your job right in the first place none of this would have happened. You were supposed to transfer my files months ago," I shot back. "This is the second time Seattle DAV has given me nothing more than a bunch of lip service. In my book, this strange idea of representation is pure incompetence."

Then I called the Seattle VA Regional Office and raised hell in the same context.

"We're sorry, Mr. Lewis, but we have received no request to transfer your files to New Jersey."

My next call was to Harry at the Newark DAV office. I told my story again.

Harry tried to sound pissed. "I personally sent in two requests to transfer your records from Seattle to New Jersey," he said. "I'll do my best to get everything straightened out. I'll find out the source of all these errors and get your records shipped immediately."

I didn't completely buy Harry's line, either.

I felt a desperate need for an independent representative who is not tied to the VA system. I am completely bogged down by a system where everything wanders from desk to desk in the same house, where everyone is everyone else's excuse-hanger and no one is accountable. I am hamstrung by the law that effectively prohibits me from getting a lawyer. I am entirely disenchanted with this country's lawmakers and its Supereme Court which legislate, enforce, and condone all these layers of inaction and ineptitude. I am in disbelief that my case is so fouled up simply because one VA doctor screwed up the original physical.

It is said that before there can be change, action, or decision, there must be a turning point. In everyday sidewalk talk you could call it a light turning on, the dawning, the last straw, or the drop that ran the bucket over. By whatever name, this day was my personal turning point. The battle line was drawn. It was now total war, me against the VA. I swear to God I am going to get these incompetent bastards if it's the last thing I do. Whatever it costs me — name, reputation, my wife ... my life — I refuse to roll over and let those morons win.

The next morning Tina came home from her shift and instantly flew into one of her rages-on-demand. Everyone at the station is talking about how I went off the deep end over a stupid letter. I am nothing but an embarrassment to her. Everything I do puts her in a bad light, nothing I do meets with her approval.

It was as if I had lost control of myself and now of my wife as well. I felt as if I was not part of her life any more.

19

Over the spring and summer a number of families moved out of the town houses and others immediately reoccupied them, and still we had not been assigned to one. Our agreement with Mrs. Thomas was that, because of the medical problem she knew I had, we would get the first one vacated.

One afternoon I went to Mrs. Thomas to discuss the matter. I fully intended to maintain a courteous reserve, to attract her with honey. But as soon as I began speaking I heated up. I wound up swearing about it, and she wound up not bothering to answer.

So I went to speak to her boss, the group commander. He said he would "check into it and get back" to me.

I didn't actually expect he would. Mrs. Thomas's husband was a retired admiral who successfully intimidated all the command. Mrs. T was about as incompetent an officer as I have ever seen, but due to her connection to the admiralty, she got away with things that would have gotten most people drummed out of the service. We are talking about no guts here at this station.

In the summer, Sandy Hook got a new commander. He was the classic example of what power does to people. He would take disciplinary action against his personnel in a heartbeat, but never commended anyone for a good job.

The commander ordered the station to quit flying the POW/MIA flag. Despite everyone's urging, he refused to fly it.
He discontinued Saturday matinees for children, which had for years been shown on Saturdays at the community center; not profitable enough, he said. He attempted to shut down the Washout Pub, presumably because it didn't fit his own teetotaling preference. Failing to get it closed, he decided to forbid senior petty officers from frequenting the pub unless it was the site of

an official station function. Apparently the commander preferred seeing his officers drive the fifteen miles to town to do their pubbing — and to drive home snockered — to their having a beer on station and then walk to their quarters.

In July a group of us went together to the Monmouth County Fair. It was a small fair, not much there, but I did find a Vietnam Veterans of America booth. The group was distributing general information to the veteran community and circulating petitions to Congress to expedite the return of, and accountability for, POW/MIAs. Naturally I signed a petition. I bought a "I Am A Veteran" pin. And I met Stumpy.

Stumpy was president of the VVA chapter; and yes, Stumpy did in fact have a peg leg, a wooden replacement for the one that was shot off in Nam. I hung out and visited with him and a fellow named Jay and the other chapter members manning the booth. I liked their attitudes about the VA, Agent Orange, and other issues that Nam vets must grapple with. These men were not nearly the radicals as the group I met in New York.

My visit was interrupted while I fulfilled my promise to take Andrea on the spins and ferris wheel, and to let her do the kiddy rides. Then Tina took Andrea to cruise the food stands while I went back to the VVA booth.

By then more members had arrived — more people behind the booth than onlookers in front of it. Stumpy, now feeling more or less acquainted with me I guess, asked me to join the group and start getting involved, right then and there. Wow ... no group had ever made me feel so at home and comfortable so immediately. Finally ... I had found people who understood what I was saying.

When I told the guys about my disabilities, the Crohn's, my headaches with the VA, everyone tossed me names and places and phone numbers to call for help. Most of the contacts were chapter members with experience in helping people with problem cases.

While Tina and Andrea cased out arts and crafts I stayed with Stumpy and Jay and the guys. (Tina would surely tally this up as six months' worth of time and attention to her little girl, and she'd no doubt claim entitlement to weeks of comp time with her drinking buddies.) We talked about veterans' issues and we rated the girls who walked by in miniskirts. If girls are going to put it on display, guys are going to look. I had a hell of a good time.

I left the group with an information packet about the VVA, copies of their local and national newsletters, and a strong invitation to join the chapter.

Andrea, worn out from the walking and excitement, conked out as soon as she got in the car. That left me to talk without distraction about my new acquaintences, and for Tina and me to agree it would be good for me to hook up with them.

"At least once a month you could connect and socialize with people with the same background and the same things in common," Tina said.

Why is it that she can be so hostile and hateful and closed to me, yet I can talk to her so freely and frankly some times?

I missed the next meeting, however, because the Crohn's had me flattened out again. I even had my ten dollars stashed. I resolved to make the next meeting, whatever it took to do it.

In August the station prepared for a *grande* celebration of the U.S. Coast Guard's birthday. There were games, prizes (I won the Fifty-Fifty drawing and collected ... *!gasp!* ... seventy-five dollars!), and activities for everyone from toddlers to great-grands. The station galley provided food, and the women's club augmented it with their potluck. A live and lively band played while we reveled the night away.

Either I got carried away with the partying or God was punishing me for having such a wonderful time, because two days later the Crohn's attacked me with a vengeance. I dropped fifteen pounds in a couple of days and was approaching serious dehydration. I was in such a bad way that Tina arranged for Christy to come "baby sit" me. Christy kept one eye on Andrea and Betsy and the other one on me.

When I couldn't even lift myself off the couch, Christy called Tina. "We've got to get that man to the hospital," I heard Christy say.

Tina apparently threw her Me First attitude under the table, because she signed off duty and got herself home within minutes. Together, Tina and Christy managed to haul me down the stairs and pour me into the car.

The hospital was in Ft. Monmouth, about twenty miles from The Hook. Every little stone in the road was a spike in my guts, and the potholes ripped them out. Little gremlins inside my stomach tied my innards into knots. This was my most painful and debilitating episode yet.

"This can't be a Crohn's attack," I told Tina between gasps of pain. "The great and mighty VA says I don't have it. It's my imagination. There is nothing wrong with me. None of this is happening."

Tina ignored me and took it for what it was: The sarcastic babbling of a bitter man in awful pain.

Tina checked me in at the emergency entrance and got me admitted right away. The emergency team performed the routine check-over, ruled out appendicitis, and called in a surgeon who concurred with my report of a Crohn's event, scheduled me for testing the next day, and immediately admitted me. The next thing I knew I was in a bed and wired up to IV's.

After yet another round of all the tests and all the pain, yet another doctor confirmed that ... (tympani ... trumpets) ... I had Crohn's disease.

I spent two weeks in the hospital.

During all that time, Tina visited me four times, ten to twenty minutes each. She never brought Andrea. Her priority was her off-duty partying. It seemed that all my wife looked forward to now was going out and getting her head bent with a bunch of teenagers; only a couple of her crew were over twenty-one.

Over the two weeks, I filled Dr. Hamilton in on the history and progression of my Crohn's, and my struggle with the Veterans Administration. Doc provided me with more information, in addition to what I already had amassed, to present to the VA. He told me he would help my case in any way he could. I said I'd advise him of my next hearing.

"There is one thing you could do right now, though, Dr. Hamilton," I said. "I could use some help in getting into proper housing at the Coast Guard station. We are currently living in an upstairs apartment with only one toilet, and since there are many days when I myself need one almost full-time, it's a real hardship on my family. The housing officer promised we would get the next available two-story, two-bathroom unit with a ground-level entrance. So far that promise has not been honored; over a dozen such units have been available, but we've been passed over each time."

The doctor composed a letter — it fell just short of being an actual prescription — and made copies for me, the base housing officer, my hospital file and all my assorted files strewn around the VA.

MEDICAL STATEMENT

> Mr. Charles Lewis, dependent of Tina Lewis, Active Duty Coast Guard, carries the diagnosis of Crohn's Disease of the terminal ileum. It would be in the best interest of his health and welfare if he could reside in housing that is on ground level, and have two bathrooms with one of the bathrooms being on ground level. Climbing stairs during the exacerbation of this disease can cause extreme discomfort.
>
> PAUL HIGHTOWER
> Captain, Medical Corps
> Chief, Internal Medicine Service

Writing this statement was considerate and generous of Dr. Paul Hightower. But was it going to be just another doctor recognizing my condition and relating it to my military duty? Would this be nothing but just one more thing for the VA to ignore and say they never saw? Why in God's name can't they just read the files, and admit that *four doctors* can not *all* be wrong? What in the fucking hell is wrong with the VA?

As soon as I got home I called Harry at the Newark Disabled American Veterans office to inquire about the status of my records, the ones he promised to assume responsibility for transferring from Seattle so he could keep his promise to settle my case.

"Oh, hi, Mr. Lewis! Your records ... just! ... arrived!" Harry said it like it was a big thrill for the world.

"Big fat overdue deal," I growled. "You said you sent the fucking request in March and it is now almost September. What the fuck do I do now? Don't tell me — I need to fill out forms. What forms do I fill out and what am I supposed to do next?"

With joy-to-the-world cheerfulness, Harry said, "You just have to wait. The *original* request that was processed in Seattle will *automatically* be addressed here."

I hadn't the foggiest notion what the hell Harry was talking about, and I bet he didn't, either. Instead of asking him to dance again with those words full of sound and signifying nothing, I said, "That's way cool, Harry, but how fucking long does it take for whatever you said happens next to happen? Do I have to wait another freaking year before I get my appointment?"

"Now, now, Chuck ... "

"Harry, I just spent two excruciating weeks in the hospital with a very major attack of a condition the VA says I do not have. Frankly, Harry, I am fed up with the VA's bullshitting around, and with the active role you have played in this whole sorry scenario."

"Now, now, Chuck ..."

"Turn the page on your script, Harry. You already read that line."

" . . . I have everything under control now. You can be assured I am doing everything I can do to get this resolved as soon as possible."

"Sure, Harry. You be sure and let me know when you've done that."

Summer wound down and it was time to send my beachcombing-and-fishing partner to the institute of formal education. We chose to enroll her in the Catholic elementary school in town. With Tina's income and my payments from the VA, I calculated we could put enough by to pay Andrea's semester's tuition in full right upfront.

But Tina had other plans for our money. So Andrea would be going to school on a month-to-month basis, budgeted from my income, which scarcely kept us in food and gasoline as it was.

20

On the evening of Friday, October 2, 1987 I finished going over Andrea's homework and allowed her to switch on the TV. I recognized the voices of Hugh Downs and Barbara Walters, the anchors for ABC-TV's newsmagazine, 20/20. I heard the words *Veterans Administration* and came to attention.

These "teaser" sound bites introduced the segment, "Whose Side Are They On?":

> "You go to the Veterans Administration and you don't know that's the enemy.
>
> "Deceit and incompetence are robbing veterans of their rights."

Quickly I grabbed a blank cassette and set my VCR to record the segment. What follows, however, is from the actual transcrip from ABC News *20/20*, air date October 2, 1987, and reprinted by permission of Devereux Chatillon and ABC-TV News. Copyright, ABC News 1987.

> WALTERS: Used and forgotten. Ever had that feeling? We hear it a lot. Some of the most frequent letters we get here at 20/20 are from veterans still coping with war injuries— sometimes unbelievable accounts of how they've been abused and insulted by the Veterans Administration.
>
> DOWNS: Yes and unfortunately, we've found evidence that if anything, their letters understate the problem — appalling cases of callous, even gross neglect of the men and women that we've

investigating the inner workings of the Veterans Administration.

JUDY BECK (wife) What's hard is when Ron was fighting out in the jungle, or any other Vietnam veteran, they fight an enemy, but they're trained to know that is their enemy; and when you come back to the States after the war, you go to the Veterans Administration and you don't know that's your enemy.

WAREHIME (a veteran): A disabled veteran in this country has no constitutional rights as far as his injuries are concerned. I'm talking about the bureaucratic system that's been set up within the Veterans Administration.

LYNN SHERR (reporter): For many wounded veterans of America's wars and their families, the wrongs begin here, at the headquarters of the Veterans Administration in Washington, D.C. As this nation's largest independent agency, it was created for one purpose:

TO CARE FOR HIM WHO SHALL HAVE BORNE THE BATTLE AND FOR HIS WIDOW AND HIS ORPHAN.

(Inscription on a plaque on VA HQ. in D.C.)
It [the VA] is the only place disabled veterans can turn for financial assistance. But there is growing evidence recently that thousands of injured veterans attempting to get fair treatment are being denied their rights by what they see as a frustrating, uncaring system.

The segment continued with Ron Beck's story.

Ron Beck served three tours of duty in Vietnam, where he earned multiple decorations for his courage and honorable service. Ron received a serious back injury that eventually left him totally disabled, even after four operations.

From the time of his discharge in 1972, he tried to get his rightful benefits and entitlements from the VA, but without success. Every time he asked for help, the VA *cut back* his benefits, until he was destitute and living in his car. That's when Ron met Judy. Eventually they married.

Judy would not accept the VA's treatment of her husband, and with Ron's agreement she reopened his claim. She included up-to-date surgeon's statements that Ron was totally disabled. But no amount of documents did any good; rather than assisting Ron, the VA simply reduced his benefits again — from $443 a month to $352. This was his only source of income.

Ron attempted to kill himself.

Judy put the VA on notice that Ron was suicidal and that he needed the benefits which the law entitled him to.

None of what Judy said or tried to do for her husband made any difference to the bureaucrats at the VA.

In January 1984 the VA sent Ron letter saying he owed the agency nearly $1800. The VA had overpaid him, the letter said, and sorry about the mistake, but we didn't catch it. If Ron didn't repay the "overpayment," the VA would stop sending his benefit checks.

> SHERR: Four months later, when his checks did stop coming, Ron Beck, disabled, depressed, and broke, took a loaded rifle to the shed behind the house and shot himself through the brain.

About three weeks after Ron's suicide, Judy Beck received a letter from the VA. The VA admitted they "made a mistake": the VA owed the Becks over $12,000 and Ron should have been getting total disability — which was what Beck had been asking for all along.

> SHERR: In one (VA Claims) office 80 percent of the cases were effectively ignored, and the file folders piled up (with no action being taken).
>
> In the Washington, D.C. office, in a blatant violation of VA rules, no evidence was regularly collected relative to document the veterans' claims.
>
> In New Orleans, claims were flatly denied, allegedly because veterans had not filed all the

> appropriate documents, even when the documents were already on file.
>
> In Pittsburgh, managers admitted they failed to notify veterans about a VA denial of their claims, thus denying the vet the chance to appeal.
>
> And some (local office) managers admitted it was their policy to deny claims before the veteran had a chance to fully develop his case, because this helped meet the established performance standards. In other words, the system rewards quantity rather than quality of work.

Then 20/20 interviewed a VA attorney. The VA does not, in fact, treat veterans fairly, the attorney said. In studying numerous cases over five years he found that the most complicated ones have the least chance of *even being handled,* because they "slow down the system" — and "most claims are complicated." More than half the veterans eligible for benefits are either denied them or simply ignored. "This makes managers look good," the attorney said.

> INTERVIEWER: By "making the system look good," what are they doing to the vets?
> ATTORNEY: They're cheating them. They're giving them a false sense that the VA's on their side, when the VA really is on the side of the people who manage they system.

Then the reporter questioned the VA General Counsel about an internal report showing the VA had a national pattern of (quoting the report) "failing to take proper action, improper development, inadequate notification and premature denials."

The VA General Counsel said he did not accept as fact, and besides, that report was two years old and "the problems have since been corrected."

The reporter produced another VA document dated less than three months before this show. (Quoting the document), "The system does not work because Regional Managers are more interested in Self Preservation — keeping their jobs — than in veterans' rights.

The VA General Counsel responded by flipping out numbers and statistics. He explained that there are "only" about two hundred fifty thousand VA employees to "provide services to about twenty-seven and a half million veterans."

(This is another instance of skewing the numbers, for this does not mean every VA employee actually services a hundred cases. Hundreds of thousands of vets' claims have either expired or the VA has let them die on the shelf, and millions more never filed any.)

One of the VA's own attorneys noted that "the pressure to make management look good" has perverted the once friendly relationship between vets and the VA. This corruption within the system is so bad that veterans need outside help to get their claims resolved. But there are two laws which prevent that help.

First, a lawyer can not charge more than $10 to represent a veteran against the VA.

The second law prohibits a veteran from suing the VA, even for arbitrary and capricious decisions or from complete inaction.

Attempts have been made over the years to get both laws rescinded, but the Veterans Administration has a stronger, better organized, more richly funded lobby than veterans have.

The 20/20 report then told of a California lawyer who, on behalf of five thousand veterans, filed a class action suit to abolish the ten-dollar limit and allow the veterans to hire an attorney to represent them. He also represented thousands of veterans exposed to nuclear radiation during and after World War II. The VA destroyed thousands of documents — records of the individuals being represented in the lawsuit.

Additionally, the VA rescinded the benefits of one veteran who was part of the California suit. This individual was exposed to nuclear radiation and was trying to get compensation for his related health problems. The VA not only denied his claim but also terminated his entitlements for the residual effects of a wartime bullet wound.

In his testimony before the House Committee on Veterans Affairs, the attorney said the (VA) system indeed needs fixing.

> DOWNS: Lynn, this is not only moving, It's Infuriating to me. I've always felt that if a man risks his life in the service of his country, we owe him a living for the rest of his life and we owe him justice.

SHERR: Well, that's what an awful lot of people feel, including a lot of veterans. These are not isolated cases, Hugh. We've heard from many, many veterans with complaints about the VA's behavior, and incidentally, regarding this court case, their behavior was so outrageous to the judge she fined the VA more than a hundred thousand dollars and appointed a special master to assure that it would never happen again. No more evidence destroyed.

DOWNS: Now if they win this case, does that mean all veterans would have the right to an attorney?

SHERR: It's not clear. At the moment, the way the case is filed, it would only concern that narrow group of veterans who have filed the suit in that class action. There are still a lot of people who believe what the veterans really need is a law passed by Congress to enable them to have lawyers.

(End 20/20 Segment)

That evening I made a promise to Ron Beck. No matter how bad things get I will not kill myself, Ron. Furthermore, in your honor, I will fight on behalf of all veterans who have been denied their benefits, and all the disabled and destitute the VA has ripped off.

And I made a pact with myself. I shall do whatever I can to make up for the betrayal of America's veterans.

I asked Stumpy and Jay and a few other guys from the VVA chapter if they had seen the 20/20 show. Most had not, but those who had watched it agreed it was a "must see" for all. So we scheduled a special chapter meeting for a showing of the video I had taped.

At the station club also, I showed the program to all who were interested. The program got the attention of most of the older Coasties; but the younger ones, the invincibles, were unimpressed, because when one is young and healthy, later-life adversities are not in the realm of possibility. Some of the senior petty officers, however, asked to borrow the video to view at home, since the station commander forbade them to go to the station club.

Tina showed no interest in viewing the program. "I can see it when we go to New York next weekend. I'm sure you plan to take it with you and sit Pops down and make him watch it."

What my wife really meant was that she didn't want to take any of her valuable socializing-with-the-guys time to share my life.

I hate New York, New York, but this time I looked forward to the trip. I couldn't wait to show the 20/20 program to the old man. So far he was incapable of believing that *H*is *G*overnment could betray its veterans. Because Pop broke an arm just prior to his scheduled ship-out to Germany during WW II, he never left Stateside. He never had occasion to deal with the VA, and being completely unacquainted with it, he adamantly denied that it could possibly be anything other than the honorable agency it once was. I will show my father-in-law the video and he will make excuses for His Government, capital letters.

On the one hand, Pop swears to the whole and entire truth of anything he sees on the TV. On the other hand, he automatically disregards anything I say. I can't wait to see his reaction to this.

As soon as Tina got off duty Friday morning she whirled into the house. "Apple City, here we come!" she chirped. She grabbed her already packed (new, spendy) suitcase. "Let's go!"

"Whoa, horses!" I said, hoping I sounded light and good-natured. "We can't go until Andrea's out of school."

"But I want to leave right now."

"For heaven's sake, Tina. All the trips we make to New York, it would be purely ridiculous to pull Andrea out of school every time we go to see your mommy and daddy."

"Okay Chuck, since you want to schedule your day your way, I'll schedule mine my way."

She disappeared into the bedroom and I heard the scritch, scritch of hangers being pushed around in the closet. Tina emerged in too few clothes and too much make-up and took off.

"So what's the use and what the hell," I mumbled to the walls and I grabbed my pole and went fishing. It wasn't nearly as much fun without my little fishing partner.

At two o'clock I went home, showered and dressed. I loaded our bags into the car, then waited as long as I possibly could for Tina to get back from wherever she was. She didn't show. I left without her to pick Andrea up at school.

Smiling and waving, Andrea skipped to the car. She expected to head straight to Grandma and Grandpa's. When she saw that her mother was absent, the child's disappointment was obvious.

"We'll pick your mother up at ... the pub." I put venom in the words and the effect was not lost on Andrea.

When I arrived and went in the revelry was in high gear and Tina was pretty mellow. "I loaded the car and picked up *your daughter*," I said. "Let's go."

"Aw, shucks, Lewis, don't rush off. Bring the kid in for a burger, stick around and join the party."

"Sure, Chuck. Couple more beers won't hurt anyone," Tina purred.

"Me? Drink and drive? With all those maniacs on the turnpike? Tina, you know me better than that."

Tina went out and returned with Andrea and sat the child at a booth. She ordered her daughter a burger, then went back to her place at the bar. I ordered an orange soda for myself.

"Orange soda!" one of the tanked-up young Coasties scoffed. "Hey, Lewis, you a party pooper or something?"

"Oh, yeah, always poopin'. Poopin's what he does best," Tina guffawed, jumping on the bandwagon of ridicule.

I took Andrea's hand and walked over to Tina and stood about three inches from her eyeballs. "Andrea and I are heading out to New York. Now. With or without you. You can get tanked up with your cronies or you can leave with us. Your choice."

The trip to the city was pretty quiet, seeing as how Tina was trying to sleep off her headache.

Just as I knew we would, we became part of the quadrillions caught in Friday afternoon quitting-time traffic. What is normally and hour and a half drive took just over three.

After supper we watched the news. Then Pop said, "Put that video on, Chuck. Let's see that show you been talking about."

"Oh, boy, Daddy!" Andrea said, all smiles. "Are we going to watch my *Incredible Journey* movie?"

"No, Honey. I'm going to show Grandpa and Grandma the 20/20 program."

"Oh, goodie! Now you watch this, Grandpa," Andrea said, snuggling in between her grandpa and grandma. "You'll see how the VA shafts people. You'll see why the guys that visit Daddy say 'the betrayal of America's veterans.' You'll see — Daddy has been telling you and Grandma the truth."

My daughter's words stunned me. I didn't know she had picked up on her grandparents' attitude about my problem. All their cloaked, patronizing remarks didn't fool even a seven-year-old kid.

I ended up showing the program twice, at their request. Walters, Downs, Sherr, et al provided the third-party information which proved the things I had been trying all this time to explain to my in-laws. When the program was over, everyone sat in silence, stunned, I think.

Finally, Pop said slowly, "I never would have thought the United States Government was capable of doing these things to those who served."

"I've been wrong, too." Tina's voice trembled. "I started thinking it was all in Chuck's head. I figured that everything that went wrong he blamed on the VA because they were a convient scapegoat."

Another turning point. At last, at long last. Bless you, Hugh Downs, Barbara Walters, and Lynn Sherr. Bless you, Ron Beck. Where I could not make them understand, you all did.

21

In mid-October the Newark VA sent a form titled "Statement in Support of Claim." It asked me to state the "problem(s) for which you wish to be evaluated." When Newark received the filled-out form they would set me up with an appointment to be ... evaluated, whatever that means.

In reference to Post-Traumatic Stress Disorder, the form wanted narratives of specific incidents and details of things that happened twenty years ago! I thought of President Reagan's response to a question asked of him at the Iran-Contra hearings: "Everybody who can remember what they were doing on August 8, 1985 please step forward." In Vietnam, wild, unexpected things happened every day, but one day blended into the next until one had no track of the name of the day or even the month.

Dutifully and truthfully, I filled out the questionnaire. However, as a preface to it, I penned my opinion:

STATEMENT IN SUPPORT OF CLAIM
VA form 21-4138

Prior to responding to this debacle I wish to make the following point.

I would like the genius who thought of this format and requirement to tell me in specific detail where they were, what they did, and whom they were with 18 years ago this date! This is an absurd requirement to place on any reasonable person, let alone someone that is in duress.

I have spent almost two decades trying to put certain events behind me; I simply do not remember all the specific details per your request.

The problem has been and still is in the overall events that I participated in. The clown requiring this information has done his job well in requiring the almost impossible from the Veterans.

I will put good money on the line that this jerk never served in the U.S. Military and is not therefore a veteran. In order to ensure a balance in the system you (the VA) continue to pit the veteran against unrealistic BS in order to present a case and prove it. This whole concept is bogus, for in most cases the veteran is dealing with people who can't identify with, let alone understand, what he has been through. Yet these same people have the authority to make decisions about veterans' lives, futures, and families.

This is just a game for your humor at the veterans' expense. So let the game begin. Keep in mind I can recreate the overall event; however, the specific details you require may not be within the realm of my recollection.

So either be serious or drop all this shit right now. This will not be easy for me, and I refuse to be led on for the sake of your humor and the hours you need to put in for the justification of your paycheck. Besides, you have access to the various military historical files.

Then I filled in the blanks, telling about "the mental antagonism that disrupted your life," or "caused you to take a different perspective about life's daily events." Then I affixed this closing statement.

After about fifteen years of being ostracized by American society, a memorial gets erected and the President says enough is enough, that we must now treat the Vietnam veterans as patriots who served their country. We must put past hostility aside and make these citizens a part of our society again. Now everything is supposed to be hunky-dory. Bullshit.

After fifteen years of being spit on — literally and actually — and considered something less than a third class citizen, I still retain suspicion and resentment. Where does this country get off trying to turn my emotions on and off like a light switch? Throw me away, then bring the decomposing person back with a piece of granite and an "Oops, sorry; let's all join hands now" — and then you have the gall to ask me why I feel I am mentally weirded out on this society.

In some ways, what occurred in Vietnam was minor compared to what happened to us after we came home. And surprise! the BS is still going on. The Vietnam vet still can't get a fair shake from the government, the VA, and yes, from much of American society. You have kept me down so long I don't know how to get back up. That is okay I guess, because you still don't know how to do your part, either. It is so much convenient to ignore me and hope that, like the good soldier, I will just fade away.

I refuse to fade away. I will continue to fight you and your system until you get off your self-righteous ass and do what's right.

On November 16, 1987, after six years and ten months, the VA gave me my first physical examination for post traumatic stress disorder and Crohn's disease.

Reporting to the Newark regional office, I took with me everything I had. The X-rays from Ft. Monmouth and the recent test results confirming Crohn's disease, all the documents and everything else from 1979 to the present.

First, the shrink interviewed me. Tell me about any counseling you have gone through. What things were getting to you now? Have you ever completed X, Y, or Z psychological tests?

I told him about the shrink-testing in Oregon, when the psychiatrist diagnosed me with PTSD and noted I should be getting disability for it.

The psychiatrist in Newark looked through my records. "I find no information about PTSD in here, nor any indication you have undergone testing for the condition," he told me. "I'll ask the VA in White City to send me a copy of your file. Then I can make a final decision about your case."

Then we got into recent and current things that were bothering me, and I was actually grateful for the chance to talk things out.

"It's pretty obvious that the disruption of your life caused by the Crohn's disease contributes significantly to your psychological problems, and so does the constant conflict with the VA," said the shrink. "The Crohn's should certainly have been identified as service connected at the very outset, but I can not and I won't go on record with that. But I am confident that will be identified and recorded when you have your medical examination here today."

The head doctor said he was concerned about the extent to which living at the Coast Guard station was affecting me. "There's too great an opportunity for you to relate things there to what you saw and did in Vietnam," he said.

"After fighting in a war, a person relates everything to the war, no matter which war and no matter where he goes afterward," I corrected him. "Maybe it's worse with Nam vets, because nobody liked the war and nobody liked the men who fought in it."

I had grown uneasy with the conversational turn and with my perceived lack of connection with this fellow. I had important things to tell him but couldn't find the words. The PTSD claim was important, but I had expected, mistakenly, that the PTSD evaluation and — I thought — diagnosis done in White City would carry the weight of that portion of my claim; I thought that part of it was pretty much a done deal. Even so, to me, the PTSD issue was not as critical as getting the Crohn's problem resolved.

In the medical department waiting room, I mentally rehearsed — again — every possible question and answer I could anticipate. I was certain that today was do or die. For the hundredth time I checked my briefcase, making sure for one more last time that I had every document, letter, report, test result, X-ray, and note I had ever received or generated about my history with this damned disease. I felt certain I was totally prepared for this examination, silently thanking all the guys at the VVA chapter who stopped by to check documents and rehearse me in preparation for this.

In twenty minutes the doctor came out to ask me to wait a few more minutes while he reviewed my claim and my medical files. A half hour passed. Another forty-five minutes. I was past worried and beyond jittery. Then the doctor reappeared and called me into his office.

This was it! The moment I had fought for ... for over six years.

The doctor didn't burn any time or calories with *Nice fall we're having* or the loaded-gun question, *And how are we feeling today?* He got right to the point, and the point was like the end of a bayonet.

"Mr. Lewis, I want you to understand that I really want to help you. But. I can't find any supporting documentation in your records in reference to Crohn's disease."

"Well, doctor, that doesn't surprise me at all. I have copies of everything that *should* be in the file you have there. But before I show them to you I would like to look through my records with you."

I had grown certain that my records had been purged by the bastards, or just as probably, documents had never been put in the file in the first place; but I was ready for that with my own papers. The 20/20 show prepared me for this, and as I sat down I said a silent *Thank you* to all the people responsible for getting that show on the air.

The doctor and I went through my entire medical file, page by page. He was right: Nothing in my records indicated any kind of digestive tract problems.

Then I noticed a manila envelope attached to the back cover of my file. "That envelope. What's in it?" I asked.

"Shouldn't be anything except routing information used by the VA."

"Routing information? What a delightful oxymoron!" I quipped. "The VA never routes anything anywhere, even under Congressional order." I thought of Congressman Elliott, but it was a story too long to bother telling the doctor. "Let's take a look anyway, doc."

The doc opened the envelope and there in front of him was ... all the information pertaining to my Crohn's disease. A report of my first hospitalization in 1980, and clearly written on it was: *"Diagnosis: Colitis or Crohn's Disease."*

I stared at the papers. "I can figure out a couple of things here," I said, thinking aloud. "Maybe this critical information was hidden away where the VA *hoped* nobody would happen to find it. But if it ever came to accountability time they could *say* it was here all along."

No response. The doc was being professional.

"The thing that's obvious, though, is: This is supposedly 'routing information.' Washington, D.C. claims to have routed my records to Seattle to send to Klamath Falls to send to New York to send to Seattle to send to Newark. Yet nobody in the history of the universe claims to have ever seen any evidence or mention of Crohn's disease in my VA file. That means nobody ever opened any 'routing information' envelope. Therefore, my file has never been routed from Washington, D.C. to Seattle to New York to Seattle to Klamath Falls to Newark — the VA never sent my records *any*where."

"This case history, all the way from 1981, puts a whole different light on your claim," the doctor said thoughtfully. I guessed he hadn't heard any of my soliloquy; his own think-wheels were turning. "Now let's put this information together, item by item, and see what we can come up with and certify your claim."

My emotions were on the top end of a bungee jump.

I presented my current medical records with diagnoses, X-rays, and the report on the upper GI series which clearly identified the site and progression of the Crohn's.

"What is your current status with the Crohn's disease, Mr. Lewis?"

I told him of my hospitalization in August and of the various episodes since.

"Are you currently on medication?"

"Thirty milligrams of Prednisone, a thousand of Azulfidine, and a vitamin and mineral supplement. The doctor at Ft. Monmouth is going to wean me down on the Prednisone after I stabilize. I have another appointment next week."

"Be sure you keep that appointment. Prednisone is a dangerous drug, and you are on a high level of it. Radiologist evaluation?"

I had it, and I handed it over.

"You came in here really prepared, didn't you Mr. Lewis?"

"I have everything you need to make my case loophole-proof."

"It says here you have not worked since March of '86. Why is that?"

"Employers won't deal with my inconsistent work habits caused by the Crohn's flare-ups. They don't like the number of sick days I take, and they don't like paying me for spending so much time in the bathroom when I do report for work. I have taken every kind of job that came along; nothing is too menial or too entry level. But nothing lasts long."

Then came the physical exam, the poking, prodding, punching, and the inevitable lecture about smoking. The doc assured me he would note that my unemployability is a direct result of the Crohn's.

At the clinic's checkout station I was sent to the cashier's station, where I was handed cold cash to cover the expense of making the trip. This was a surprise; I had never before been reimbursed for any VA-mandated travel. The sum I received more than paid for my gas ... but I parted with almost all of it just getting my car out of the parking lot. In a city like Newark, where parking is such a premium, gas is only a secondary expense.

When I got home I called Stumpy to tell him I could almost smell success at last. Next I checked in with Christy, who by prior arrangement was already planning to pick up Andrea after school. Then I headed straight to the club.

Roger, off duty from the station shop and on duty behind the bar, nodded and drew me a draft. Roger was Tina's first line supervisor. He was an okay type of guy, but one of those petty officers who had no concept of military leadership. He knew I thought so, for we had many a heated discussion. Somewhere in the course of them, I usually told him how buggered up his attitude of leadership was, and he told me how buggered up I am in general. Nevertheless, we were friends. Stumpy once likened us to abused mates who kept coming back for more.

I could absolutely rely on Roger for two things. A generous beer. And to pass around everything he heard. Roger and his wife Christy were ... let's say they networked. Therefore, I told Roger the story, that I was satisfied with how everything went, and impressed with the attitude of the staff at that particular VA office. The Newark VA staff was cordial and helpful from the moment I walked in until I left. Finally ... a professionally conducted office of the Veterans Administration.

"I really really really hope everything gets straightened out by Christmas so I can finally do something special for Tina and my kid," I told Roger. I knew Tina would hear that direct quote right from Roger, and that was fine; I wanted her to know she was still first in my heart and first on my list.

"Well, buddy, congratulations. Twice. Once for the good news, and once for not blowing the whole deal by exploding on them. I know you were, as you said, prepared to go to war with them if need be. To tell you the truth, Chuck, a lot of guys were waiting for a news bulletin about a veteran going off the deep end and trashing the Newark VA office."

It was a slow evening at the pub and Roger and I frittered away the evening schmoozing and mini-bowling and ... well, getting along, for once.

Tina stopped by the club and picked up some sodas and munchies for the evening watch.

I stood beside her as she studied the snack department. "Guess what? Things went really well at the VA. For a change."

She picked some items and I followed her to the cashier's.

"We should have some word about the first of the year."

She took her change, acknowledged me with a curt nod of her head, and walked out.

The next morning, when she got home from her shift, Tina finally asked about my visit to the VA. *As if she hasn't heard all about it by now.*

"Well, you can expect nothing to happen again. As usual."

Gee, thanks for your loving uplifting supportive optimism. "Yes," I acknowledged. "We sure know better than to count on the earth to move for us. But you know what, Babe: I really feel positive about this go-around."

I extended the strong arm of hope, but I could not force her to grasp it. But I ... I would not let go. It is said that when a man has no hope, he has nothing. I refuse to be left with nothing.

High hopes put me in high spirits, and that put me into the holiday mood early. The station began to buzz with plans for the annual Christmas dinner dance. It was to be a formal military ball; I had attended a number of them in the past and I loved them! I was pumped for this one, excited to be attending one again. I hadn't taken my wife to a dress-up affair in a very long time, and it was important to me to show her a good time.

I couldn't possibly swing a nice dress for Tina and a suit for me. So I opted to rent a suit and spend every nickel I could afford on her. I wanted her to look like the demurely elegant lady

I married, not like a grunge-dressed bimbo out beering with the boys and not like a station grease monkey.

We went to Monmouth Mall and invaded all the more-up-scale women's shops. We chose a royal blue satin gown that made her look like a queen. God, that woman was a beautiful sight to behold. A knock out. A refined vixen. Oh, but I was going to be proud to escort my wife to that dance and show the morons at the station what a class couple looked like in a civilized social function that went beyond the standard beer bust.

We finished our shopping and got back in time to pick our daughter up at school. Andrea was thrilled to have her mother pick her up. Sadly, that happened only rarely.

With Thanksgiving, Hanukkah, Christmas, New Years Eve and New Years Day coming up, it would be a draw of the straw as to what holidays everyone would have off. Tina, being a new non-rate without any position, would probably get stuck with duty on most of them. Holiday duty schedules had been turned in to the station commander, but he was being his normal asinine self and not making his decision known until the last possible minute.

The commander completely ignored the schedules composed by department heads and made up his own. Tina got New Years off and worked Thanksgiving and Christmas and the day of the kiddies' Christmas party; it looked like the Almighty Commander deliberately scheduled all parents to be on duty during the kids' party. There really are brass-people in the military whose attitude toward family is "They knew when they signed up that duty would interfere with family, so by damn, I'm going to make sure it does."

Tina had invited her parents, her sisters and their husbands and kids, and her aunt and uncle for Thanksgiving dinner, which was a big all-hands banquet at the station. If Tina had known in advance she would be on duty that day, perhaps she would not have invited them ... Naahh. She would have anyway. The house was filled and running over, I was supposed to entertain them, and I did not want to deal with the scene. I do not do Thanksgiving very well.

On Thanksgiving Day, 1969, I lost an entire patrol of men under my command. We advanced into a booby trap. Some of my men were blown apart; most of the rest bled to death on the chopper that came to rescue us.

And the chopper's crew chief — all the while he bitched because he couldn't get to his Thanksgiving dinner until he reached the hospital and then cleaned my men's blood out of his aircraft. Here were soldiers, the dead and the dying, and all this alleged patriot could do was crab about how all the good stuff would be gone before he got back to the mess hall.

Did he want me to apologize for my men being so clumsy as to step on a mine and inconvenience his day?

This is one of our legacies of that war, that men saw so much killing and maiming and torture that they became jaded — and Americans have been jaded and unfeeling and indifferent ever since. All wars are terrible, and all take their permanent toll on the survivors. But this one was the worst, because it was an undeclared war, an unconstitutional war, and the military higher-ups never told the men in the trenches why they were there. Maybe that was because the higher-ups didn't know, either.

Now decades later, every Thanksgiving I see and feel that day in Vietnam. I see the fire and smell the smoke of that explosion, and feel the shrapnel flying past. I see blood flowing from wounds until there is no blood left to flow. I see the life fading from those once vibrant, devil-may-care youthful bodies. Nothing I can do puts the blood or life back in them. All my efforts and all my praying do not bring them back.

Thanksgiving is my personal Memorial Day for five guys who made a mistake in war. In war there is no quasi-error; there is life and death.

For Tina's people, the holidays are unwaveringly family times. They did not want to allow me my solitude. Did they think they could get me into their program just by giving me an order? "Chuck, celebrate!"*Yes, SIR!* "Chuck, be merry!"*Yes, MA'AM!*

Since our first Thanksgiving together Tina has known my feelings. I cannot help but believe that she made this occasion a set-up, another way for her to justify to everyone that I am another wacked out vet.

Naturally Tina had to put me up for public ridicule when we all showed up for dinner. She joined her father in commenting that I felt too good to join them at the dinner table.

I helped Andrea with her dinner tray and saw that she was seated and having a good time. Then I went home to be alone with my thoughts — and to allow my wife and her family the time and space to make fun of me.

By the first week of December I was antsy about the results of last month's shrink-and-physical "visit" at the VA. I called them to inquire. The response was: Wait.

Wait for what? It only takes a day for a doctor to write his report and make recommendations.

"I just wanted to know the doctors' findings."

"We can not provide that information," said the VA.

"But this is *my* claim. I ought to be entitled to information about myself."

It's happening again. Once more I'm getting fucked over.

There has to be someone out there who can help me. It isn't the Veterans Administration and it isn't the Disabled American Veterans. It isn't a congressman or a senator.

So I sent a letter to President Reagan.

Mr. President:

Sir, I am writing with the hope of obtaining some assistance with an ongoing problem with the Veterans Administration.

I provide the following background:

I served in the Army from 1968 until 1981, including two tours of duty in Vietnam.

In 1979 I contracted Crohn's Disease, an inflammatory bowel disorder, which cause is not defined. Crohn's disease requires specialized medical care and follow-up which I was not able to receive on active duty. In 1981 I therefore opted to resign my military career, planning for civilian and VA follow-up. Such has not been the case.

Crohn's disease is not covered on a civilian insurance plan because it is classified as a pre-existing chronic condition. The VA, through its offices in Washington state, Oregon, and New York, has done nothing, despite its claims to the contrary. I have received nothing but a massive run-around.

The following is only a sample of the problems I have had with the VA.

1. During the original evaluation in 1981, the proper tests required to diagnose the disease were not made. The tests I was given were not ones which detect that problem. Some of the lab work the VA claims it did was in fact never done.

2. No one in the VA explained the appeal process. The VA in Seattle did claim it sent out such instructions, but such instructions were sent to an address at which I never at any time lived.

3. The several times I sent the VA additional information about my case, it usually has conveniently been lost.

4. The VA either neglected to answer, or provided only partial answers to my questions.

5. When I compiled the necessary information for my appeal, I handcarried the packet to the VA. The counselor there informed me that it would not get approved or recognized. In other words, the request for appeal was denied by a paper-shuffling clerk. I was denied due process without the slightest consideration of facts presented. Just as a note of interest, this particular counselor was maybe 22 years old and obviously not a veteran.

It is now December 1987. I have finally received a hint of recognition from the VA here in New Jersey. On November 16, 1987, I managed to get another physical for post-traumatic stress disorder problems and the Crohn's disease.
The PTSD evaluator stated that he believed the stress disorder and the Crohn's are related. The evaluating physician stated that I have had Crohn's disease since 1979. This is two years prior to my discharge.

I find it curious that every doctor I have spoken with outside the VA in New Jersey seemed to know what and how to test for Crohn's disease. Yet as the result of incompetence at the Seattle VA, I must prove a case that should have easily been proven seven years ago.

I am unemployable, as no employer is willing to pay anyone for spending two to four hours a day in the bathroom. I have sold everything I own that is of any value. I don't even have a bed to sleep on. The soles are coming off the only pair of shoes I own. I used up our family savings a year ago. I now face another Christmas of nothing for my wife and 6-year-old daughter. I can't afford the medication I am supposed to take.

Sir, I am sick and God damned tired of all this. It still takes the VA six to 12 weeks to accomplish each step of the process, and every step so far has taken me back to Square Zero because each decision of the VA has been a denial of the rights the law supposedly allows me.

The end result is no matter how hard I try, I get nowhere. I have become a burden to my own family and I have nothing positive to look forward to in the future.

Mr. President, I am asking you to intervene if you possibly can, and push the VA along on my claim. I believe if the VA were to get serious this could be settled in a couple of weeks, thereby allowing my family to get on our feet.

If it becomes necessary to wait another six to nine months all this will be academic, because I will not be alive to see it. If nothing else my wife and daughter can claim my life insurance. I am tired of beating my head against a wall, and of being a burden to my family. I can no longer accept the system I fought for but is now turning its back on me, and on so many other veterans as well.

I implore you to exert your influence to allow the American Veteran the rights they fought to defend but are themselves denied: the right to Due Process. Legislation must be passed to allow veterans the right to take the VA to court, the right to file suit for benefits the VA denies them. There is no excuse for the VA to have strung my case out as it has. Their conduct in my case, and in hundreds of others similar to mine, is nothing short of reprehensible if not downright criminal. The Cubans in LA and Atlanta have more rights to due process, and they are criminal non-citizens.

I am not suicidal, yet one must do what one must to care for his own. Not that it matters, but the statistics speak for themselves. It's a remedy that creates one less headache for the VA. Small wonder why more Vietnam Veterans have died at their own hand than were killed in the war itself. If the VA is so righteous in the manner it operates, why is it so afraid of the veterans having the option of going to court?

I leave it to you to do whatever is in your power to assist with my case, and with the cases of thousands of other Vietnam vets as well.

Sincerely . . . .

I held no delusions that President Reagan would personally act on my behalf, nor, for that matter, that he would ever personally read my letter. But I did firmly believe that no president, nor president's staff, since John F. Kennedy really understood veterans or knew what went on behind the closed doors of the VA; it is as anonymous as the IRS. I also believed in planting seeds: I believed that whoever on Reagan's staff read my letter (if anyone did) might begin to realize some changes need to be made. I had no delusions, either, that any changes would come about in the next year or three ... but who knows; if the VA gets overhauled and if Vietnam vets' rights get recognized in ten or fifteen years, perhaps my letter to the President carried one of those seeds.

22

By the second week of December I still had not heard from the VA. Since that august agency had scarcely ever moved a molecule without being prodded (and since the waiting was driving me nuts), I placed a call to Newark.

The phone was answered with the predictable greeting: "Please hold for the next available counselor."

After please holding for five minutes, a counselor picked up and said, "Good morning. May I put you on hold?"

It wasn't exactly *hold*. It was *ignore*. The lad didn't push the hold button; he merely set the phone on the desk. I spent twenty-two minutes, prime-time toll call, listening to the Civil Servants' Party Planning Commission.

"So whose party we going to tonight? We gotta make some decisions here."

"Al serves good drugs."

"Ben has the horniest women."

"Cal seems to have a decent mix of both. Fair stuff and okay broads."

"So where're we gonna go?"

"We could take our own hootch and our own dope and go for the hottest chicks."

"Why do we need to pay for quality when we can get medium-grade for free?"

"Well, we gotta decide where to go and if we're gonna take stuff or just freeload."

So much for the government's war on drugs.

Finally, "Okay, make the list. I gotta catch my cust — " Scritch of phone as it's being picked up. "Oh, shit."

The oath meant the clown on the line noticed he hadn't punched the "hold" button. Now he realized the office chatter had been heard, and the damage done, because when I asked him his name he would not tell me.

"Okay, that's all right," I said. I identified myself, gave my case number, and asked about the status of my case and my appeal.

I heard papers shuffle. Then, "I can't find anything here or pending."

"I would like to speak with a supervisor, please."

The party-minded VA clerk would not transfer my call to a supervisor, nor give me a phone number. This is a direct violation of VA policy.

Finally the party boy just hung up on me.

I called again and again, and every time the person answering the phone refused to speak to me or refer me to anyone who could help. It was as if a message had gone out instructing everyone to have no communication with me.

I poured another cup of coffee and tried to figure out how to get to a supervisor.

Then I remembered that government office structures use consecutive blocks of phone numbers. 555-5555, 555-5556, 555-5557. So I should be able to dial the next higher number and get another office that might transfer my call to a supervisor. On the third try I dialed directly to the supervisor's office.

Yes, this was indeed a supervisor speaking.

I introduced myself and stated that I wished to file a complaint about an employee under this supervisor.

"Wait a minute, Mr. Whodidyousay. How did you get my phone number? Clients are not supposed to have supervisor's direct numbers. Who gave you this number? This is directly counter to instructions here."

This is great. This so-called supervisor doesn't want to hear about employees who are more interested in drugs and booze than in doing their job. He wanted the clerk's ass because a veteran got through to him on the phone.

Hey, Chuck. Who do you s'poze decides whether a supervisor is doing his job? Who do you s'poze evaluates the evaluators? Yes, this guy must be involved in drugs himself, or else he's sticking his head in the sand because he doesn't want to deal with personnel problems. *He doesn't want to deal with a veteran's problems, either.*

This guy babbled on and on. "How did you get my phone number you are not supposed to have access to this number you aren't supposed to call me. ... " So I interrupted.

"Excuse me, sir, I didn't get your name." He hadn't told me and I didn't expect he would now. He didn't.

Then I proceeded to articulate my complaint about the clerk who kept me on hold while he discussed his party plans.

"First I'll look into finding out how you got this phone number, then I'll look into your complaint," said the supervisor. "But you'll have to put it in writing." To his credit, he did tell me the correct mailing address to file my complaint. But it was obvious he wouldn't do anything about it.

"Thank you, Mr. Supervisor. I am sincerely thankful for your interest in my case and in my future, and I appreciate that you will look into the misconduct of your staff. I am cognizant of the difficulty of your situation and I thank you for your conscientiousness." I hung up and basked a little in my Academy Award-winning pretense of warmhearted gratitude.

In reality I wasn't feeling kindly at all. The urge to go to Newark and totally wipe out the VA once again grabbed me. Just blow up the entire building and send them all to fire and brimstone.

What is scary is this is only one incident in one small branch of this country's bureaucracy.

I called Stumpy and told him the latest installment in the VA story.

"Not surprised at all," Stumpy said. "Nothing those guys do surprises me any more."

I said, "It isn't just a matter of protecting the constitutional rights of a government employee to fry his brains and pickle his liver. It's protecting the rights of those the servants are paid to serve. The ACLUers demand the civil servants' right to stay stoned, and the rest of us wind up relinquishing our right to a decent society. Whenever one screws off, someone else gets screwed over. And veterans are in the hands of the screw-offs."

"Tell ya the truth, Chuck, I think they set out to rile and frustrate. Vets get disgusted and quit trying to deal with them, and that works out real well for the government. It lowers the VA's workload, and it saves the government money."

"I'm going to send a formal letter of complaint," I said.

"Probably be a waste of your stamp, but you should do it anyway. It'd take a million complaints to shake up the system, but yours could be the millionth."

As I saw it, part of the problem is the flagrant attitude many government employees have toward those they are supposed to be assisting. The VA is staffed by people who have never been in the military, never faced an enemy paid to kill them. They have no understanding of the military, of combat, and of life thereafter.

Veterans would be better served — hell, they would be served at all — if veterans manned the VA system. There are enough disenfranchised veterans, some of them already educated and some needing training, who could fill most VA slots. Veterans understand veterans in a way non-veterans never will. They understand the real problems involved ... and they can also pick out those trying to B.S. the system.

It can be argued that the President makes a major effort to place a distinguished veteran activist in charge of the VA, but that is meaningless when the person in charge hasn't the power to fire incompetent employees because their job is protected by the civil service union. And no matter how dedicated, energetic, dedicated, ethical, or competent he is, no single individual among thousands of employees can fix such a corrupt system.

We must return to supervisors the power to fire the incompetent, and there must be a higher supervisor overlooking their actions as well. The politics of it is that Civil Service workers' union wouldn't allow Congress to strip the union of its power to protect the incompetent jerks who receive paychecks while they plan parties and make drug deals on taxpayer time.

Think of this: Every American dealing with the government, whether it's the VA, a tax auditor, student, building inspector, or whomever, could be putting his finances and his personal life in the hands of druggies and hustlers. Every government employee should be subject to random drug testing, and those testing positive should be fired immediately, no administrative leave with pay or anything else that keeps the paycheck flowing into the drug network.

I mailed the letter to the regional office that afternoon. I knew it would be buried and ignored, and that nothing more would come of the issue.

Now I needed to get my mind on something more positive, like the upcoming dinner dance.

It was the first social event I had really looked forward to in years. For once I wanted to have a good time ... and to show off my beautiful wife.

The day before the event Tina came home from work and dropped her bomb on me.

"Chuck, your presence is not wanted at the party."

"What do you mean, I am not wanted."

"Just what I said. Several individuals put the word out that it would be best for everyone if you weren't there."

"Who said so? Why?"

"I'm not going to name names. But several people made it perfectly clear that you are not wanted."

"Okay. All right. We'll just go out somewhere else."

"No, Chuck, it doesn't work that way. Everyone is looking for me to be there, except without you. So do me a favor and don't make make a big deal of this. And for God's sake please don't make an issue of this around the station."

"Wait a fucking minute. You are planning to attend this little charade and leave me home? Will you tell me what the hell is really going on?"

"Nothing is going on. You are just not wanted. I am. I'm going and you're going to stay here with Andrea. You can save the babysitter fees, since you're always bitching about our money situation."

I had just been kicked in the head.

I went to the beach to walk and think.

In my head I knew that things were just about over between us, but in my heart I wanted to keep my family together.

Raging, I blamed the VA. For stripping me of my status of breadwinner and head of the household. For forcing me onto welfare. For forcing us to have to live with her parents, my parents. The VA forced us into homelessness. For forcing my wife to join the Coast Guard because I was unemployable, and she resented both me and the Coast Guard for that. She was furious with the VA with its endless supply of loopholes to hide behind, and that made her furious with me.

I hated and despised the VA. Damn, I wanted to kill everyone involved in that system.

The day after the dance, as I wandered the compound, a dozen times or so guys stopped to ask why I wasn't at the dance. "It was a total bore," some said. "Wish you'd've been there to liven things up."

My friend Tim hailed me down and invited me up to his apartment to have coffee and warm up.

"Surprised to see you out on this chilly morning, Chuck," he said. "Everyone thought you were sick again 'cause you weren't at the big do last night."

I told him why I didn't go.

Three days later I met up with Tim at the station post office, and he pulled me aside to talk.

"Chuck, I spent a couple of days checking out Tina's story about the dance. I talked with practically everyone at the station and not a single person told Tina you weren't welcome. Looks like you were lied to, my friend."

I mulled a moment, then said, "Tim, I have no idea why Tina does what she does, and it would be useless to fight it out for an explanation. The good news is finding out I'm in good grace with the rest of the station. I thank the messenger for that."

On December 16, 1987 I received the report on my physical. After almost seven years, the VA finally got around to admitting I had Crohn's disease. I was awarded a disability rating of thirty percent, effective March 1987. I would receive a check for the amount of my retroactive entitlement "in the near future."

Now the door was open for me to pursue my case for retroactive benefits back to 1981, and seek a one hundred percent rating due to unemployability. These points could have been addressed as being integral to the rating, and should have been. Perhaps this was the VA's stab at trying to economize. They may have tossed me a slice instead of the whole loaf, hoping I wouldn't notice being bilked out of seventy percent of my rightful entitlement.

The stress disorder was not addressed at all. I wondered if Newark was having trouble getting the information from White City, Oregon. I wondered if Newark had bothered to ask, or if Newark asked and Oregon didn't bother to send it, or if the VA was simply too pea-brained to be able to consider more than one subject at a time.

"I've heard the VA uses that piecemeal approach on a regular basis," Stumpy said when I told him about it. "It's nothing other than a delaying tactic. Unfortunately, most vets take what they can get and quit out of frustration."

The evening of the day I actually received the money from the VA we had a small celebration at the club. Roger was running the bar, and made sure the beer kept flowing. As people came in during the course of the evening, Roger made sure they knew I had scored a victory.

Tina, on duty that night, came by to pick up some sodas to drink at the station. She glowed in the congratulations being heaped on us for putting up a winning fight. She acted as if it weren't for her nothing would have been accomplished. Still trying to be the center of attention.

"Thank you thankyou. ... I just kept urging and supporting Chuck. ... He'd talk about giving up and I wouldn't let him."

Tina cozied up to me at the bar and gave me a big hug and a kiss. That took me by surprise; it was practically a miracle happening. Well, if one miracle can happen, maybe two can, and I had visions of things being the way the used to be for us. Then she bought a half rack of beer and was out the door ... and the only vision left was the one of her and her duty section getting tanked up again.

Tina returned from duty Friday morning hand out, palm open. "Give me your VA check so I can buy Christmas gifts for my family."

"Can't. It's gone. I paid up our household bills and Andrea's tuition." *And I cached some cash for Andrea's Christmas, but I won't tell you about that or you'll find it and spend it all on some brat-nephew who has no priority whatsoever in our lives.*

This year Tina cleaned us out (again) and plunged us into debt (again) with trinkety extravagances for her family, and foolish splurges for herself. By my own armchair analysis, my wife had a pathological need to put up an appearance. She wanted to fulfill every impulse right now; "plan" and "wait" were concepts beyond her narrow gasp.

One day I analyzed "the Tina situation" and realized her reckless, selfish spending was not her only maladjustment. All of her own shortcomings she loudly attributed to my stress disorder problem. Wigged-out vet, she told her buddies; you've no idea how hard it is to put up with / stay sane around / leave my child with a wigged-out vet. My few close friends said the only problem they saw was Tina.

Of course she managed and manipulated the youngsters on her shift. She was charming and charismatic, and the 18- to 20-year-old kids were easily suckered into believing her lies.

We spent New Years with her family. Naturally. I hoped for two things: To spend New Years Eve with my wife. To talk to her parents about getting her some professional help.

After supper Tina's sisters announced they and their husbands were going to visit some old school friends and invited Tina along.

"I really want to go, Chuck, but I'm afraid you'd be out of place with Sis's friends. You and Andrea stay here and have a good time with Mama and Pop. We'll be back in an hour or so."

"An hour, not much more," Tina's brother-in-law cut in. "I'll personally see to it."

At seven-thirty they left, chattering and giggling.

Being left out was a crushing disappointment. And excruciatingly humiliating, being rebuffed in front of my wife's entire family. But, oh well, it was also an opportune time to try to talk to Tina's parents. So after Andrea went to bed at eight-thirty, I told Mom and Pop about Tina's recent shenanigans, concluding with my concern for her need of professional psychological counseling.

"Tina is a sweet, gentle, considerate person," said her mother. "She would never do those things."

"Nope, you're the one with the psychological problems," said Pop. "You see everything all skewed."

"Well, you're seeing one 'for instance' right now. It's ten o'clock. She's an hour and a half late and nobody's called with an explanation. Based on the stunts she's been pulling the last six years, she won't be back until well after midnight."

"No way," Pop snapped. "She says she'll be back in an hour, she'll be back in an hour. Two hours, most. Come on, Mama, let's go to bed."

I waited up, alternately reading, coffeeing, and wandering outside in front of the building, catching a little fresh air — or as fresh as it gets in the midst of New York City. At ten to six I decided to catch a few winks. Just as I started to stretch out on the couch, Tina and her entourage came in.

"Good evening and morning, Tina. What happened to the 'I'll be gone an hour then we can go do something for New Years Eve'?"

"Don't jump on her, Chuck," Tina's brother-in-law chimed in. "It's not her fault; I was the one driv —"

"Shut your face while you still have one, you little I'll-personally-get-her-back-in-an-hour." I came *this close* to beating the hell out of the little shit.

"Shut your own face, Chuck!" Tina hollered. "I can party with anyone I please. Anyone would be more fun than you!"

"Well, thank you for all your consideration. Why in hell didn't you at least have the courtesy to call? For all we knew you were lying somewhere bleeding to death — this is the Big Rotten Apple, you know."

The uproar awoke Tina's parents. Her dad jumped into it.

"She doesn't have to call and she doesn't have to justify a damn thing to you, you wacko. Next thing you're going to be making up lies about your wife 'going off and doing her own thing' or some other crazy paranoid thing."

The pressure building inside me was about to boil over. Either I explode in violence, or . . .

I picked up my overnight bag. I picked up the sleeping Andrea, nightshirt, blankie, and all. I carried her down to the car.

"What are you doing?" Tina screamed, staggering out behind me.

"Going back to The Hook."

"Without me? How am I going to get back?" she cried.

"I really don't care." I unlocked the car and gently lay Andrea in the back seat. Then I got in and started the car.

Tina came running to the car and jumped in as I started to pull out. She was raising hell about my leaving without her.

"Andrea is being neglected and I am not wanted here. We are going home. Now. I have no intention of spending another minute in this mess." I was out of the parking lot and on my way.

"My stuff. My nice clothes. You can't drive off and leave all my things!" Tina wailed.

"The only clothes you need, lady, are uniforms and jeans for housework. I'll let you out here and you can go back and get your junk, but someone else can take you home because I will be gone. And when they do bring you home, tell them not to get out because as long as you and I still live in the same house, your family is no longer welcome in my presence."

I pulled over to the curb so Tina could get out, and waited in suspense to see if she would.

Tina buckled up and settled back in her seat. "Let's go," she whispered.

"I don't want another word out of you," I said. "Andrea's having a hard enough time with all this shit."

Our little girl was wise to what was going on, but confused about her mother's conduct. She asked me more than once why Mommy didn't do anything with us any more, and why she wasn't home when she was off duty. The one that hurt the most was when Andrea asked why Mommy had to go out and get drunk with all the guys. Tina couldn't even hide her conduct from a seven-year-old.

When we arrived home Tina jumped out and went straight to the station, New Years Eve clothes, hangover, and all. About ten o'clock in the evening she came in, grabbed her uniforms and make-up kit and left, without so much as a word to me or Andrea.

After totally avoiding Andrea and me for nearly a week, Tina came home again. The New Years incident was apparently behind us; everything seemed to be back to normal. Better, even. Perhaps Tina had taken the event as a lesson.

The next evening we went to the club for a couple of beers. The only ones there were the kids that Tina worked with, all of them well on their way to sloshdom. She ambled to their pushed-together tables and sat. I spent two hours sitting alone while she played her little games with the kids. No lesson learned at all.

Every damned one of them drooled over her, flirting, using crude language, even touching. I couldn't take any more of it so I tried to get her to come home with me. But she decided to stay with the boys. I cannot describe the total humiliation of being tossed into a corner while my wife flipped herself around like a common bar tramp.

I worried about the frequency and amount of Tina's drinking. But more than that, her whole duty section's drinking habits constituted a serious breach of national security, as far as I was concerned. At least four of the men-children were known as problem drinkers, and the rest were willing participants, never mind they were underage. Some even sipped on duty. The command structure knew, and turned a blind eye. Another fine example of Coast Guard leadership.

Here's a scenario for taxpayer cogitation. A ship in distress, hundreds of lives at stake. Or enemy ships approaching the Eastern Seaboard. The United States Coast Guard, ready to defend and protect. Except the unit supposedly ready to protect is plastered. They're incapable of even boarding their patrol boat, much less rescuing and defending.

There comes a time when when we vets must swallow our feelings and get away from the stressor, If we do not, we explode and add fuel to the stereotype we already carry. I was not going to give these youngsters the satisfaction of exploding in their presence. None of them was worth the effort of a good ass kicking.

I left Tina with the children, just as she had commanded me to do, and I went home.

23

At home I watched the late news, then folded out the couch and made up our bed.

Tina slithered in about midnight and eased into bed.

I tried putting my arm around her. She kicked and turned away. Then she inhaled and tuned up.

She raved about how I couldn't get work, that if it weren't for her we would be on welfare. Which was true, but I didn't ask for this disease and I was going out at least once a week looking for work. Even the guys in the VVA chapter who worked for the New Jersey Department of Labor couldn't find me any work.

Then she started in about how I couldn't go out socially without worrying about having an accident in my pants, how I wouldn't get farther than a few steps from the nearest toilet, how I am messing up *her* life with my medical problem.

That was the truth, but when we married we promised to love each other in sickness and health.

"And another thing ..." Tina shrilled.

I knew from years of experience that when Tina said that, she was getting cranked up for an abusive tirade.

". . . You're just letting the VA jerk you around. You're in a dream world if you expect them to actually change your files. The VA is probably right, you don't have all those so-called entitlements. You're a bum looking for a free ride, just another fucked up vet who can't get along with people. You can't get the VA to support you, so you're using me."

She went on. And on. About how I ruined her life, interfered with her independence, wasn't fit to be in her presence, and she didn't like the way I danced. She reminded me of every little thing that ever went wrong in our lives, our plans, our marriage.

Then she dropped the big bomb on me.

"The whole reason I joined the Coast Guard was so I could be independent and support myself and kick you out of my life. I'll tell you what, Chuck: I deserve a hell of a lot better than you. But I do appreciate your sticking around to take care of Andrea while I work my way up."

Tina didn't touch me, but I felt like she'd ground a high-heeled shoe into my balls.

I exploded. "Hey, listen, honey baby independent self-supporting boy-chasing wife. I have a perfect solution to your fucking problem."

It took but a millisecond to jump from bed to closet and grab the thirty-two caliber automatic pistol and draw it from its holster.

She sat on the bed, cheering me on with eyes that screamed, "Do it. Do it and get it over with."

In one smooth motion I pulled the slide back and locked and loaded the chamber, clicked the safety off, and placed the gun behing my right ear. I felt the trigger give and the locking mechanism of the hammer start to release, preparing to blow my life, my disease, and all my frustration and confusion straight to hell. Flashing through my mind was the thought that I was about to do the VA a big favor by eliminating another problem they didn't want to deal with.

For that moment I was a blank spot in a nether space, an unperson. Neither alive nor dead. No pain, no hurt, no laughter, no elation. No feeling. Just a serene sense of quiet existence, a being without physical senses. A non entity occupying space and time.

Events of the years raced past my mind's eye. I saw a military career fold because of an incurable disease the VA said I didn't have. Felt the chaotic return from an unpopular war. Felt the stinging hostility of the American people my leaders said I was defending. Recalled a beautiful, loving wife. Saw the birth of a wonderful daughter. Watched a man crushed and a marriage crumble because of a damndable disease.

I saw a promising, new found civilian career disappear, literally, in the toilet. Pride was no longer my personal descriptor, dignity a thing of the past. The very government I served and dedicated my life to now turned its back on me.

My mind replayed the words of a United States Congressman telling me and thousands of other veterans that we and our service meant nothing. That the Constitution we swore to defend didn't apply to us, that we were third class citizens without the rights which that Constitution bestowed on everyone else.

And my mind printed a picture of a man I had only seen on a TV screen.

Just as I felt the hammer on the pistol start to let go, reality hit me. Who the hell did this bitch think she was, and what in hell made her so fucking special? I would be rolling over for the VA and letting them close the books on my case the easy way. And poor little Andrea, she would spend her life thinking the father she adored was a quitter.

But most of all I would be failing in my pact with Ron Beck. I never even thought it crazy to have a pact with a dead person I never knew ... but in sense that was real to me, I did know Ron Beck. I made a deal in his honor. No; no, I will not dishonor him by backing out of that deal.

"WHY? GOD DAMN IT ALL, WHY? SOMEBODY ... ANYBODY ... PLEASE HELP ME."

Slowly I lowered the pistol and returned to the living. I shook violently despite the balmy evening. I unloaded the pistol, throw it back into the recesses of the dark closet and slammed the door shut.

Then I went to room where my daughter slept, looking on her beautiful innocence. *May you never know how close you came to losing your father forever.*

I took my jacket off its hanger. Tina, my once adoring wife no longer existed as I passed her on my way out the door. In the moments just unfolded, she did and said nothing except for her comment when I picked up the gun: "I hope you don't make a big mess."

I am convinced that she had long been planning to push me to the point of no return. Yes, it is clear now. She planned to rid herself of me and she didn't care how it happened. All she wanted was to be able to present the pitiful wife image to her family and friends. A divorce was such a despicable option, it would hurt her image.

I walked away from the building which held my unhappiness, searching for solace in the night air and the rippling of the incoming tide beating its rhythmic cadence on the rock jetty.

As I approached the jetty of the bay at Sandy Hook, New Jersey, I thought of how my life had been turned into such a dismal state. Was there something or someone to blame, or was it all my own undoing? Is this self-pity ... or is it injustice? I just don't know anymore. All I know is that my disability has been ignored by the agency that is supposed to care and compensate. Or am I crying the blues to justify my own shortcomings?

Or am I a classic example of the indifference of the Veterans Administration?

Suddenly, a voice from nowhere ... from everywhere: "FIGHT."

"Yes!" I answer. I am right, and the system is wrong. Someone has to take the stand somewhere and at some time. I can not lose; I have nothing else to lose. Yes, I will fight — I must. I have never rolled over for anyone or anything in my life; why start now?

I am not crazy. Yes, I am ill. But yes, I can still get justice. Not just for myself, but for all my brothers and sisters who have been betrayed by the government we were once so proud to serve.

I must pull myself together and get focused. All right, first point: My marriage is over. Right now it is no more than a mutual convenience. I need the medical care I can get as Tina's dependent until I finish my fight with the VA. She needs me for a housekeeper and handyman and babysitter until she comes up with a promotion with self-supporting pay.

Second point, I must rededicate myself to winning my battle with the VA. A settlement, and the retroactive entitlements I am owed, will enable to me get custody of Andrea. I will start all over from the beginning, if I have to, with truth and facts in hand. I will force feed it all to them until they either choke on it or admit their errors. I must out-persist the VA. I cannot blink, and I have to be willing to bang my head against the ivory tower of the VA and its strange concept of fairness and justice.

I wandered along the jetty and breakwater until four in the morning. The gentle *lapple, lapple, sshhhh* of the tidewater washing against the jetty cast a soothing, tranquil effect on my raw nerves. The skyline of New York City at dawn made a splendorous facade for our most corrupt example of government and man's inhumanity to man. Yet on this particular night there was serenity in the silhouetted city. I could hear the low murmur of engines of the ferry taking the local yuppies to Manhattan for another day's work.

I let my mind drift to mellower places and happier times. An occasional splash of a jumping fish or an acrobatic sea bird would bring me back to reality and put me on edge again. For a long time I drifted from a peaceful blur to the edge, but not, this time, over it.

24

When I returned home just after four in the morning, Tina was up. She had been busy: her bag was packed. She was literally moving in at the station.

"I'll be back when it's time to pack for Petaluma," she said. Then she left, she just left, without so much as a good-bye to Andrea. If I were a hard-nosed, conservative judge I would call it child desertion, and that's why I entered the event in my journal. I doubted that Tina had a prayer of getting custody of Andrea when we divorced.

We saw nothing of Andrea's mother until it was time for her to leave for California.

Back in August Tina decided she wanted to attend the Coast Guard's Emergency Medical Technician training course in Petaluma, California. She had been a medic in the Army and she was a good one. She had the background, and she had the inborn ability that would make her an excellent EMT — if she felt like working at it. The training would help her with the much needed promotion points required for advancement. It was only a three-week course, and, as I told Tina when she first mentioned the possibility of attending, Andrea and I would miss her but we'd get through it.

So in August she applied, in November she received her acceptance, and now, in January, she was on her way to California.

All the way to the airport, Tina kept quiet except to tell Andrea that she would write to her and call her regularly.

"Oh, goody, Mommy! Send me cards with pictures of California! I can show them to the kids at school, and then I'll put them up in my bedroom."

Just before Tina boarded, Andrea hugged her mother, long and hard. "I'm going to miss you, Mommy," she said.

For half a year now Tina had spent very little time at home, and scarcely any one-on-one time with Andrea, anyway. Whether she was holed up at the station or across the continent would make little difference in the amount of time she spent with her daughter. I wondered whether our daughter would actually *miss* her, or if she was merely expressing her insecurity about her mother's constant absence from her life.

Tina was true to herself. She never called Andrea or even sent her a card. She had time to tour the wine country and send letters to her station cronies telling them about it, but her own child never got the first note. I devoted myself giving my daughter a rich and great time while Tina was gone.

Tina came home three weeks later with her Emergency Medical Technician's certification. Andrea had shown no pangs of separation, no melancholy in her mother's absence, but when Tina walked off the plane and scooped Andrea up, the child was as excited and happy as a rescued puppy.

"You go claim my bags," Tina ordered me. "I'm going to talk with Joe over there. He was at EMT school with me."

"To hell with that shit. I'll wait for you to talk, then we'll go to baggage claim."

"To hell with *you*, Chuck, you controlling son of a bitch. Nothing's changed with you, I see."

No, nothing's changed. It looks like nothing ever will. I sighed, but I stood my ground and waited while Tina talked to her newfound ... buddy? Was he just a military buddy?

Damn it all, I really did want to salvage this marriage. *Why, Lewis? Why would you want to stay married to her, after all she's done to you?* Because I love my family and I want to keep it together. Go away, Voice.

Winter melted into spring and activities started to pick up at the Vietnam Veterans of America chapter. The unit was invited to march in a community's annual St. Patrick's Day parade — the biggest parade on the Jersey shore. From the founding of our chapter its members had been in this parade. It allowed the public to say thank you to Vietnam vets; for many of them, it was the only thanks they ever got.

I had reservations about putting myself in that parade. I was nervous about admitting to the public that I was a Nam vet. I had been shamed and ridiculed enough for my role in that segment of American history. Despite "public opinion," I am proud that I went when I was called, and grateful that I survived multiple tours of duty. I am proud that I didn't duck out by hiding in the halls of ivy or running off to Canada or to "study" in England. Regardless of my personal disagreement with the war and our reasons for getting into it, I am proud that I didn't fail my country or my brothers in arms. I was there, and I didn't hide behind a bunch of pretenses. I accepted the challenge and I paid the price, and that gives me the right to speak out when I see things I believe are wrong.

Nevertheless, I wasn't ready to walk in that parade. Each vet has to decide when he has healed and ready to come out of his shell, but it's an individual matter for each man.

In late winter local schools invited chapter members into their classrooms to talk about Vietnam. I told the VVA members about Seattle's very successful classroom program, Vietnam Veterans Leadership Program.

"Kids today need to know and understand what happened during and after that miserable debacle," I told my VVA brothers. "Their history texts tell 'all about Vietnam' in two paragraphs. If the kids get any more than that, it's always the anti-war, anti-authority, anti-patriotism, flower child point of view. It is obvious that the *"historians"* don't want to use facts and the whole story," I spieled.

"We have an obligation to educate, because nobody else seems willing to tell kids the truth," I kept spieling. "If we don't, then young America will forever believe the revisionist crap they're being fed now — that we should apologize for Hiroshima, Stalin was a nice friendly chap, there is no such thing as post traumatic stress disorder, that the best and brightest went to Canada or England instead of Vietnam, and the Holocaust never happened.

"We're supposed to learn from our mistakes. But you have to know what the truth is before you can tell what the mistakes are. Not the Hollywood theatrics but the real truth. Students must learn the mistakes of history or be doomed to repeat them. It is important that we" — with both arms I gestured to include every man in the room — "speak of our expernences so the students understand."

The upshot was: I was elected to coordinate all the speaking programs in the schools. The number of chapter members who volunteered to participate was overwhelming and gratifying.

With each presentation our program became more refined. We developed a pretty good mobile musem of "show and tell" items of personal memorabilia. We discussed each aspect of the war, from the initial French occupation to our own escalation, to TET of 1968, Agent Orange, the anti-war protests, and the aftermath of the war and how "The Sixties" changed our culture.

Talking to the kids was totally delightful. They asked thoughtful questions. They thanked us — they actually came to us after class to thank us for coming into their classrooms.

We started something that will be an important contribution to education in our area, and to our community. It felt good to be part of such a program.

Despite all that was happening in my personal life, which was rapidly falling apart, I continued my quest for work. I made an appointment with the VA Vocational Rehabilitation program.

On April 22, 1988 I reported to the Newark VA Regional Office. In careful detail, I explained my situation to the counselor.

"Your best option is to file for a federal job," he told me. "Your disability rating gives you preference for any job you are qualified for. Our program could also send you to school . . . Let's see here ... " He ruffled through my file, looked at my college records. "Nope, not necessary; you already have an Associate degree. You have plenty of experience and education to qualify for a good position."

The sun was rising on me again.

The counselor gave me the usual and expectable bundle of papers to take home, fill out, and return. He photocopied my current papers which showed a 60% disability rating, directed me to the desk where I should obtain a Letter of Certification declaring my disability rating and a Civil Service Preference form, and made an appointment to return and hand over all the papers he required.

At the front desk I showed the papers I was supposed to show, picked up the papers I was supposed to take, and hurried to get to Andrea's school in time to pick her up.

At home, while Andrea poured over her homework I looked over my newest armload of papers. The Federal Application Form — My god it was long. Asked for a hell of a lot of information. Filling this one out would be no fifteen minute job.

The Civil Service Preference letter from the regional office — I opened it, read it and reread it. I refused to believe what I held in my hand.

CIVIL SERVICE PREFERENCE

The following certificate is furnished for your use in establishing Civil Service Preference.

This is to certify that the record of the Veterans Administration disclose that **Charles A. Lewis** is in receipt of disability compensation on account of service-connected disability rated at

~~(30 percent or more)~~ (less than 30 percent)

This payment is made in accordance with public laws administered by the Veterans Administration.

Marsha Jones
Veteran Service Officer

The ignorant fool who completed this form marked the wrong block. The last time I checked, sixty percent was *(more than)* thirty percent! God almighty damned, these fucking morons can't even underline the proper words on one paper while holding the information in the other.

My God, I gave the stupid broad a current copy of my disability rating — the one the counselor upstairs photocopied so everyone had the latest, accurate information. She also could have checked the VA computer system to validate it. Now how in hell can she turn around and underline "less than 30 percent"?

Worse still, Ms. Marsha Jones is a department supervisor. The supervisor did not check the accuracy of what she signed; hell, maybe she didn't even look to see *what* she signed. Well, the stupid bitch is probably a "preference" hire and she can't read anyway. God, for all I know, the stupid bitch was one of the druggies who wound up *not* helping me in December.

My ammunition against the VA is growing. If we vets ever get the right to go to court, I'll have these bastards squirming all the way to the unemployment line. One of these days that sorry agency will get exposed, and I will laugh while they fry.

Okay, okay, it's partly my fault. I should have looked at the paper before I left. Okay, it's not Armageddon. Next week, when I turn in my Federal Job Application (the employment people say it in capital-letters), I will get the error corrected. My anger wasn't that the mistake couldn't be rectified, but that there was no excuse for ever having made it.

That evening I showed this Civil Service Preference to some guys at the club. After the initial shock, everyone tried cloaking their hostility in black humor ... drugged-out bureaucrats, subnormals in government, business as usual. All-around, overall SNAFU. As one fellow said, "Government agencies are equal opportunity offices ... Every citizen gets equally fucked over."

On March 27 I went back to Newark for my follow-up appointments. The first place went was to the main office to get the Civil Service Preference Form corrected. As soon as I walked in I knew this was going to be a grim session: Some twenty men were awaiting their turns.

The person who marked the wrong block on my form was at the reception desk and Miz Supervisor Marsha Jones who signed the incorrect form was busy-motioning around in her office at the rear of the room. *Lucky day, Lewis. With all the players here, this will be a minor little thirty-five-second matter.* "What do you want?" the clerk snapped snapped.

Oooo. She's having a bad day! Well, it's about to get worse.

"Excuse your attitude," I said. "I am here to have you correct a mistake you made on my Civil Service Preference Form.

"I have never seen you before. I have no idea what you are talking about. Sign in and have a seat. You'll be called in the order you signed in. Forty-five minutes to an hour."

"I don't have time to wait around because I have an appointment upstairs in fifteen minutes."

"Well, sir, I'm not the one who scheduled it. Please have a seat and we'll call you in turn."

"Look, lady, I waited my turn last time and if you hadn't fucked up this simple little form then I wouldn't be in your ugly face right now. This is a pre-printed form and all you have to do is type in my name and underline the correct statement. Since the one you underlined is the incorrect one, it shouldn't stress your cranial capacity much to figure out how to fix it."

If she had projected a pleasanter attitude when I approached her, things would be going in a different direction right now. But she turned my crank, and I wasn't going to be bluffed.

She look past my left ear and eye-contacted the guy behind me, and, pretending I was not there, she spoke to him. "What can I do for you today, sir? I'm here to help you."

Nodding toward me, the fellow said, "This gentleman's ahead of me. I can wait."

"Ma'am," I said, coating my tone with fake sugar. "All you need to do is cross out four wrong words and underline four right ones. Or you could start over, type two words and underline four. If you had done that when I asked you to, I would already be out of here. I realize you are in charge of this desk at this moment; but, Hon, snarling at people, denying that a mistake was made, and refusing to rectify that mistake are not effective ways of being in charge."

I knocked the sugar off and got emphatic. "Now, lady, I have not read your job description, but I bet that somewhere in it is a hint about serving veterans. It would be very nice if you could do that once in a while and ..." I raised my voice another two notches ... "STOP YOUR BULLSHIT EXCUSES. Now will you please get this form filled out properly so I get the hell out before I really get pissed."

By now the other ladies behind the counters had been sent to this bitch's aid. Supervisor Jones never left her office. All men working at the United States Veterans Administration were huddled together in a corner about twenty feet from the counter.

Security came in and tried to clear everyone from the vicinity of the counter but I didn't back off. "You aren't chasing me out so easily," I said loudly. I decided I may as well speak up so everyone could hear, because everyone witnessing this incident was bound to talk about it afterward. I didn't want anyone misquoting me because he hadn't heard me clearly.

"I am totally fed up with the constant incompetence of this fine organization and I am not moving until Miss Dingbat corrects her fuck-up. If dip shit here will make the damned correction I will be gone. If that is too much to ask, then we can fight if you want, and I won't mind explaining to the judge why I'm arrested.

"Yeah, you security forces, come to think of it, that would be a good idea. Let's just go and explain to the judge how veterans are treated like shit whenever they walk through the doors of this building."

One of the women had taken my Preference Form from Miz Dip's desk, made the correction, and handed it to me.

Our eyes met. I read the apology in hers. "Thank you for your twelve and a half seconds of giving a damn," I told her, and I hope she saw in my eyes that I meant it.

The Voc Rehab people were waiting for me. I handed in all the papers, including the corected Civil Service Preference. Then I told the counselor what I went through to get a correct copy.

All he said was, "Yeah."

"So that's pretty much SOP, huh?"

The counselor shrugged and made an eyebrow and a mouth that said, "Well, you know how it is."

"Any preference as to type of work you want?" he asked.

"I would take anything I could get. If I had a list to choose from, though, I really want to put my engineering skills to use. Because of the Crohn's, I need an office job with an absolute minimum of field work. The Sandy Hook-Ft. Monmouth area would be convenient, but I'll go anywhere in commuting distance."

Concluding the interview, the counselor said, "I'll distribute your application everywhere. With your qualifications and education, I'm confident you'll be working within weeks."

Part of it was a pep talk the man is paid to give, I figured. People were being laid off at Ft. Monmouth and at the weapons yard at the Earle Navy Station across the bay from The Hook. But I grabbed a pocketful of the counselor's optimism and I hurried home to start waiting.

25

My Vietnam Veterans of America chapter received invitations to march in several Memorial Day parades. I decided that I was finally ready to walk in a parade, but hadn't made up my mind which one. Tina's good fortune decided for me.

Tina was selected to be in Highland City Memorial Day parade. She would ride on the station's LARK, an amphibious vehicle used when local roads flooded in rainstorms or hurricanes. I no longer had to agonize over my own parade-day decisions. I preferred taking Andrea to see her mom in a parade. My daughter and I had a great time planning how we'd have a great time — cheer Mommy when she goes by, see all the displays, eat a ton of junk food.

On parade day, Tina had to report for inspection and formation, so she left the house long before Andrea and I.
I decided to wear my jungle shirt with my awards and other stuff. It was my silent announcement that I am a veteran, and this day was special to me.

Andrea and I got to Highland City about ten-thirty and went straight to the American Legion Hall. Phil, a Coastie at The Hook, was tending bar and Andrea and I sauntered up and had a seat. Phil drew a Coke for Andrea and a beer for me, and she felt pretty big-timer, sitting at the bar and drinking with her daddy.

A number of legion members were in the club, and Phil introduced me around. Most were vets of Korea, some of WW II, and a half-dozen members were Nam vets. We all chatted a while, then the chapter commander invited Andrea and me to walk in the parade as the chapter's guests. So the two of us and the American Legion commander led the parade.

I think Andrea had the day of her young life. Leading the parade, marching beside her dad. Smiling and waving to the crowd. She saw some of her schoolmates and hollered and waved. Well, *they'll* spread the word, I thought, and tomorrow every kid in her school will know Andrea was in the parade!

I was having such a good time watching my daughter that I forgot to think of myself or my fears or to be self-conscious.

Then a lady ran out of the crowd and grabbed me. She gave me a hug and a quick kiss on the cheek. "Thank you for what you did for your country," she said. She ran back to the sidewalk and disappeared into the crowd that lined the street.

I cannot adequately articulate the emotions of that tiny speck of time it took that woman to do what she did. This was the first time I had ever heard those words, the first time in over seventeen years anyone said thank you for serving.

Thank you. Just a simple thank you; that's all any of us wanted. We never expected everyone to fall at our feet, we just wanted some acceptance, and the right to resume our roles in our country and communities.

A light switch had clicked on inside me. Suddenly I was proud of who and what I was.

Now Andrea knew for a positive fact she was right: This whole parade was for her and her daddy. Truthfully, I felt the same. This parade to honor our fallen brothers was the welcome home I never got. It awakened my sense of pride. I was a person again. Part of society. I had just been accepted. The world was not out to get me because I served my country.

I now regretted I had not done this before. Stumpy was right. Getting out and getting into the world helped break the chains that bound us to the bitter part of the past.

After the parade Tina rounded us up at the Legion Hall, where they were serving free hot dogs and drinks to parade participants. She got a dog and a soda and pulled up a chair beside Andrea. *Look at you guys, Lewis. You're being like a real family. Hot dogs and pop after the Memorial Day parade.*

"Can't stay; have to drive the vehicle and crew back to the station," Tina said. She turned to Andrea. "Want to ride the LARK with me, honey?"

Andrea's eyes sparkled as she gave her mom a wide smile and vigorous nod. Riding a military rig driven by her mom ... what a capper to the day!

Tina said she'd get a sitter for Andrea and come back and join me.

I stayed at the Legion Hall and socialized with everyone and had a hell of a good time. One after another, Legionnaires struck up conversations with me, and each asked me to join the chapter. I was honored. And greatful, appreciative, and renewed. Nevertheless, I knew the deep-down, underlying, real reason my membership was so much wanted. The local Legion chapter, like Legion chapters throughout America, was dying, figuratively and literally.

Tens of thousands of vets returning from Vietnam attempted to join groups like the Legion and Veterans of Foreign Wars. But those organizations didn't recognize Vietnam as a "real" war. "The enemy" did not pose a direct threat to American soil or American people. Few Americans understood why we were there (including many of our troops and a fair number of our military brass). Congress never declared war; therefore, those who said our being there was unconstitutional had an arguable position. For those reasons, plus all the reasons of individual, personal prejudices, we Nam vets were not welcomed into membership in the Legion, VFW, DAV, et al.

Historically, veterans have had considerable political clout, principally through their veterans' service organizations. They contribute money to candidates and testimony to committees. But since Vietnam vets didn't count with those organizations, the fraternities didn't speak on Viet vets' behalf. Neither the veterans' organizations nor the Congress supported Vietnam veteran issues.

But earth circles, time passes, and guess what: All those World War Two heroes began fading away and those Korean vets began aging and the veterans' organizations began to realize they were endangered. During the eighties, local chapters all across the country began disbanding and closing. So the fraternaties started courting Vietnam vets. If a family line is to continue, it must produce a next generation, and all of a sudden the older vets decided they were just kidding, bring your money and come perpetuate the organizational family name.

Veterans' organizations have enormous potential for delivering service and education to communities, and for gaining benefits, good PR, and political clout for their members. But all potential good gets diluted or lost because of provicialism and infighting among groups and leaders. Veterans are losing entitlements at an astounding rate and the only way we can regain them is to unite our voices. We have got to stop the infighting as to which organization best represents the American veteran, and whose war was the worst or more real. It's easy to blame Congressional inaction when veterans lose their rights; it's obvious to rage against the VA when vets are not served. But Washington will be allowed to continue its negligences until the leaders of the various vets' groups stop squabbling among themselves and get on with the issues at hand.

I told the Legion commander I would be at the next chapter meeting. In the meantime, I had some serious drinking to do.

My money was not good that day and evening at the Legion Hall. For the first time since arriving at Sandy Hook, I was awash in friends — and they all set me up one. I wasn't stupid-drunk, but I sure as hell felt good.

Tina never showed up. I called home but got no answer. So I sipped and chatted a couple more hours before I gave up on her and headed out. I wasn't sloshed, but I had no business driving.

At the station, Washout Pub was obviously an alive and hopping being. Full parking low, and above the din of the crowd rose the thunk-boom-tootle of a live and lively band. Something was up and I figured Tina was being a part of it. I parked the car at home and hoofed it to the Washout Pub.

What was happening was the Park Rangers' end-of-the-volleyball-season party. Nearly all the patrons were Parkies, very few Coasties. Packed club, good band, and me, still in party mode. And Roger's familiar face behind the bar.

"Hey, man. Good shirt. Never saw you in your Army togs before. Great jewelry you got there." He tapped some ribbons on my chest.

"Hey, Roj. Walked at the head of the parade over in Highland, me and Andrea. Boy, is this a memorable Memorial Day. Set me up a couplea suds, Roj."

From the tap Roger filled two frosted mugs and set them before me. Then he stepped back two heel clicks, and saluted. "These. Are. On. Me. SIR!"

About ten-thirty Tina came in. As she came to the bar I gave her a hug and asked her to dance.

Her response was to grab my shirt sleeve and pull me outside.

"What the hell's the idea, not waiting for me to go get you? I wanted you to stay put until I got there."

"Well, Tina, you left at one-thirty and I waited around until quarter to ten. You said you'd be back in, quote, *about an hour.* How in the hell long was I supposed to wait?"

Then Tina went into a rage about me driving myself home after all my drinking. She had no way of knowing how much I had to drink — she was right, but her method of assessing the truth was wrong.

"You're right. I apologize for that, Hon. Now, being as we're here, let's go in and party."

"I don't want you to go back in there, Chuck. You're not wanted. The only place you're going is home."

"Sorry, Tina. If I go home, you're going with me. If you want to stay and party, I stay and party with you. I'm going back in the club now, and I'm going to keep on having a good time until you make up your mind what you want to do."

One of the Parkies had just bought another round when Tina came in, in a total rage.

She fumed that I was an embarrassment and she was fed up with my shit. I still had on that "theatrical" jungle shirt with my decorations, which looked stupid now that the parade's over. I was intimidating everyone and they can't enjoy themselves when I'm here.

"Tell you what I'll do, Queen. My presence seems to stir up your pathological temper. I'll leave so the party doesn't get ruined because of you."

"Good. Leave. Roger, give me a wine cooler and charge it to Harrison over there." She took her drink to a table occupied by Coasties. It looked like Tina had a whole new squadron of buddies, because none of the guys at that table were ones she worked with.

I was not ready to leave, and by God I was not going to. I stayed at the bar.

"Who put the bug up her ass?" a Parky wondered.

"I didn't notice *him* being any problem. She is, though," said another.

"Yeah, but he sure *has* a problem — her." said a third.

In about ten minutes Tina stomped to the bar raising hell again about why I hadn't left.

This time I talked some sense into her and she decided to go home with me. All this time the two Parkies beside me were being careful to look like they weren't listening while they carefully listened. I was sure the Lewises' spat would be widely, told, retold, and mistold in the next few days.

The next morning Tina made a half-assed apology. "What got me going is that you had no business driving home."

"I acknowledge that. But why didn't you come get me, like you said you would?

"Because you were enjoying yourself and I wanted to give you time to have your fun."

She means she lined up some fun on the side for herself, and she didn't want you in the way.

I let her know that her misconduct in public of late is uncalled for, and I would not accept that kind of conduct ever again. Those scenes have got to stop.

It is clear to me that she was playing mind games. She wanted to get me to believe all problems are my fault. She wanted to make me believe there was nothing wrong or immoral about her behavior, that the only thing wrong was me; I have PTSD. Well, she was the one looking foolish; she is the one losing the war of wills, because I won't take her bait.

The next day Tim and I met for our scheduled rendezvous at the fishing bank. Immediately, he started bawling me out about the scene *I* supposedly created at the club last night. "Word is out that you got wigged-out and everyone was afraid you were going to beat the hell out of Tina right then and there."

"Where the hell did you hear that?" I demanded.

"The guys she works with."

"Tim, none of those kids were at the club last night. So you tell me — where did they get that piece-of-shit story from?"

So. She was still trying to make her cronies think I was the wigged-out Vietnammer. Poor, suffering, unappreciated, misunderstood, abused wife. I was starting to put two and two together, and it kept coming up Tina.

Suddenly Tim saw the same picture. "Holy shit, Chuck! She is really doing a number on you at the station. What in hell is her problem, anyway?"

We changed the subject to Tim's upcoming wedding. He was getting married in December and we were all going to participate. Tina was going to be a bridesmaid, Andrea the flower girl, and I, Tim's best man.

After Tim left I reflected on Memorial Day. Wasn't it curious that the United States Coast Guard Station, Sandy Hook, New Jersey did not hold even a brief, simple ceremony for Memorial Day? And curiouser, nothing at all for Veterans Day? Nor National POW/MIA Recognition Day. It was galling enough when the new Station Commander ordered the POW/MIA flag should no longer be flown; but it was reprehensible when he refused to unfurl it on National POW/MIA Recognition Day.

Practicing the principle that nothing ever gets done unless someone does something, I wrote a letter to the Group Commander. As a branch of the Armed Forces and the U.S. Department of Transportation, I wrote, the base should rightly hold at least a short ceremony on commemorative days to recognize those who served. I would be happy to plan and produce any future ceremonies in the event the station hadn't the time or personnel for such a project. I proposed spearheading activites for POW/MIA Recognition Day and Veterans Day.

The Group Commander met with me to discuss my proposal. He thanked me for my interest and input and said he would recommend to the Station Commander that I organize those observances.

26

The women of Sandy Hook organized a ladies softball team. Tina joined the team and I helped with the skills coaching. After two or three weeks of not very serious practice, the team was about to embark on its first game. It was us versus Ft. Monmouth.

Our team was just terrible! In their drubbing-in-progress, the women became increasingly agitated, bad-attituded, and their playing, which started out in the pit, went downhill from there. I tried to coach, to talk to them, but the team's head coach sent me to a spot far outside the diamond. The Sandy Hook girls got their clocks cleaned fifteen to three.

After the game the women gathered at the Washout Pub. There I found out why I was kept off the diamond, and why the women were so distracted. Tina's teammates had been unmercifully harassed by Ft. Monmouth's male fans. Catcalls, inuendoes, sexual crudities, degredations, and propositions, and overall downright filth. The girls kept me out of earshot because they were scared that I might try to take out the vulgar ones. They were right about that.

"Why didn't your coach complain to the officials? Why didn't your teammates' husbands do anything about it?"

"Our men didn't know what to do. They didn't want to cause any problems. Besides there were a lot more on their side than ours."

"Why in the world didn't you just walk off the field?" I asked.

Stoic answer: "We were determined to play out the game. We decided we ... would ... NOT ... be ... run off the field."

I know for a fact that conduct like that is not accepted and not allowed in the military. Yet those Monmouth men are in the service, and so are the husbands of The Hook's team. How did it come to such disregard, then such wimpy tolerance?

Despite my problems with Tina, she was still my wife and I was not about to take this incident lightly.

I suggested the women of The Hook's team write a letter to the Station Commander and ask him to file a complaint and protest on behalf of all the ladies at Sandy Hook. It was decided that two team members would meet with me tomorrow to put together a good letter. After everyone signed it, Tina would present it to the Station Commander.

I also planned to call in a formal complaint the first thing in the morning.

First I called the sports department at Ft. Monmouth. The guy adopted a "so what" attitude and blew off the whole incident. And Tina, who was home for a change and heard my end of the call, bitched at me for "getting hostile." Hell, she's soantagonistic toward everything I do, she gets angry when I try to stand up for her. I don't think she even noticed that I was the only husband willing to walk the plank to try to get this kind of stuff stopped. Or maybe she thought that since she was so liberated, she could handle the crudest vulgarities but didn't know what to do with gentlemanly behavior.

Next I called the Ft. Monmouth chapter commander's office and talked with the deputy commander. "Be assured I will get to the bottom of the situation, and corrective action will be taken," he said.

The pair of teammates who volunteered for letter-writing patrol showed up and we composed our letter to the Station Commander.

> On 6 June 88, at 1700 hrs. at Ft. Monmouth field #2, the Women's Softball League played its first game of the season. We played the 174th MI Co. Team #2b, and believe it, it was an experience we did not expect.
>
> Our Coast Guard and Sandy Hook women were subjected to explicit sexual and racial harassment. The following are only some of many examples of statements and actions directed to us by the men of Ft. Monmouth.
>
> 1) Ref. CPO Cleary's wife: "Send her fat ass back to Puerto Rico." (She is Samoan.)

2) Several women were called "Whores looking for a quick fuck after the game."

3) "Coastie dyke who can't play on dry land."

4) Blunt statements referring to team members' anatomy that were not only insulting but totally abhorrent.

5) Women sliding into base were told "That's where you belong, on your knees ready to give a head job."

There were many, many other such comments from the Ft. Monmouth male coaches and spectators. The language and conduct of their team and spectators is not only counter to the wholesome spirit of the game, but it can be classified as child abuse because it occurred in the presence of dependent children out to watch their mothers play ball. Such conduct is also illegal according to United States military regulations.

I am proud to report that even under such trying circumstances our ladies maintained their dignity, pride, and sense of good sportsmanship. However, we will not tolerate such demeaning ridicule in the future.

We respectfully request that you lodge a formal complaint in support of our ladies team and demand an immediate apology to our team.

The duo took the letter to their teammates and all but three or four were available to sign it. The next morning Tina took the letter to present to the Station Commander.

That afternoon I happened to meet up with the Group Commander. He knew there had been a game, but he was stunned when I told him what had happened. "Tell Tina I would like to endorse your complaint to the Station Commander," he said. I relayed the message, and Tina said she would ask the Station Commander to pass the letter to the Group Commander for endorsement.

The Ft. Monmouth Deputy Commander retuned my call, just as he said he would. "You are right to file a complaint, Mr. Lewis.

I have taken action against all guilty parties with an official reprimand in their records. I am particularly saddended and disgusted that one of the offenders is an officer. Now, sir, may I speak with your wife, so I can personally apologize to her on behalf of this command?"

I exlained that she was on duty until Monday. The deputy said he would like to contact her at the station office. I gave him the number, and we hung up.

I appreciated the Deputy Commander's phone call and his apology, and felt confident he meant to deal with the perpetrators. I had no idea if he planned to talk to the Station Commander or not, but didn't particularly care. I got my satisfaction.

When I went to pick up the mail that afternoon I stopped to see if Tina had given the letter to the Station Commander, and to ask if the deputy commander contacted her. As soon as I walked into the shop Tina jumped on me.

"Go home and bring back a needle and thread so I can sew your mouth shut. Also bring back the typewriter so I can throw it in the bay."

"Meaning what?"

"The Station Commander got your little proposal about pomp and pompous ceremonies and he didn't like the plan at all. He also has no intention of interfering with the women's softball league. He suggests, and I quote, 'If you can't take the heat, get out of the fire.' What he meant, dear Charles, is: If women in the military can't take care of themselves, quit the team."

Then she said, "Wait, there's more. Fort Monmouth Sporting Department called the Sandy Hook Commander complaining that a husband from the Hook had threatened violence at the next game. Guess what, Charles — the commander figured out it was you. Imagine that! You are so famously well known around here, even the commander thinks of you first when someone goes ballistic. Anyway, our commander is a bit pissed at you. It would be smart if you stay away from here for a while."

Everyone had gathered around by now, including Tim, who is my friend; he is also Tina's supervisor, too, remember.

Tina began laughing. "It's all a big hoot, Chuck. It's funny, don't you see? So what do you think about that?"

I thought plenty.

I thought it was very sad when a military installation does

not see fit to observe important military occasions. Maybe the commander was angered because he thought I was being critical, or maybe I stepped on his inflated ego.

I thought our Station Commander was terrified of anyone who outranks him, and he would rather not speak up for the women of The Hook than face his superior officers.

I thought nobody at Sandy Hook and nobody at Ft. Monmouth had the guts to speak up about anything, not even to protest the degradation of their wives.

All I said to Tina's crew was, "I think a man who will not take to task anyone who insults or defiles the woman he loves is an uncaring wimp. I think a commander who will not defend and back up those in his command is a coward not worthy to command. Tell me you'd like to go into combat with a leader like that."

Tim, who is normally pretty cool-headed and who's the one on that crew with the most sense, spoke up. "So now, Tina, you see what your commander thinks of the ladies out here. He's sexist. Pleading your cause to him is a waste of time."

"But you got an apology from Ft. Monmouth, Tina," I said. "At least *one* officer is a gentleman."

Tina relayed a message from the Station Commander that if I had anything to say to him he wanted me to say it face to face, not through a letter to the Group Commander.

All right, face to face was fine with me. I called the station office for an appointment with the SC. Finally, after some run-arounds and avoidances the yeoman on duty (who happened to be Tim's fiancee), reported to me. "The Station Commander said he couldn't see you for two weeks." No surprise there.

In the meantime the SC was doing a hell of a job making Tina's life miserable. This SC was just plain vindictive, but beyond that, he had no clue about basic human relationships let alone any regard for regulations. But Tina, not one to take flak from anyone, had an investigation launched into the SC's conduct. After determining that she had a case to bring charges against him, she told him she would hold off, provided he ceased his harassment and left her to do her job.

A few days after filing the letter, I happened to see the Group Commander. He commented that he was still waiting for word from the SC because he was eager to add his endorsement.

I showed up at the appointed time. The station's executive officer was present at the meeting because the SC would not see me alone. *He's nervous and agitated. Good.*

"First off, the only holidays I recognize at this station are Christmas, Easter, and Coast Guard Day," said the SC.

"Why? Why not Veterans Day and Memorial Day? Why not Armed Forced Day and Independence Day?"

"If I celebrated them then I have to let all the Nig ... I mean Blacks celebrate Martin Luther King Day."

Let it go. File it in your mind and use his racism against him another day.

"I don't quite understand, Sir. What does Christmas have to do with the military? Are you referring to the events of Valley Forge or something?"

"I don't know what you mean about Valley Forge, Mr. Lewis."

So this high ranking military leader knows nothing of military history. He probably thinks the American Revolution is some new kind of ferris wheel.

He tapdanced through a few tirades, and I let him tap. This was his station and everyone in it will do what he wants. He was a religious man and there would be no observances where people expect beer. The POW/MIA flag would not, repeat *not* be flown at this military installation "as long as I am the Commander here and that is final, and I don't care about any state laws."

Then the SC let me know that the station did, too, in fact have a Memorial Day ceremony. Yeah, I heard about it. It was a sermon on the evils of drinking and driving, and boating without a lifejacket. Probably closing with a prayer by the minister of whatever church the SC was prostelyzing.

"Sir, there are a fair number of Vietnam veterans on this station, as well as some from the Korean conflict. Veterans Day, Memorial Day, and Flag Day are times to respect and thank *all* veterans of *all* wars."

"I have no problems with veterans. After all, I am one, myself ... "

Veteran? Of what? Officer Training School? His uniform bears a few Attaboy ribbons, and not even the National Defense Service Ribbon.

" ... but I am not about to get overly worried about a bunch of men who have nothing better to do than go to a meeting and cry about their war experiences and swap psychological symptoms over stale beer and loud music."

Now it was time for a new tantrum on a new subject. As far as the vile behavior of his men and of the men of Ft. Monmouth ... well, boys will be boys, it's just a little wholesome, good-natured razzing; and girls who can't take it can leave. "And you, Mr. Lewis, have no business interfering with station command and policies." And no, if it were Mr. SC's wife, he would not intervene. If women wanted to play with the boys, they can't come running for help when they think the rules are too tough.

I burst out laughing. "You mean to tell me, sir, that the vile and disgusting comments made to the ladies of your command meet with your approval as wholesome razzing? You mean you find this okay as a man, a husband, father, commander, and a religious person?"

He railed on and on about sexual and racial harassment not being that at all. Then, "Let me tell you something, Mr. Lewis. I have not taken any action on your wife's request to intervene. It is not my policy to get involved in these trivial things."

And in conclusion, "Mr. Lewis, you are not to go to any more games of the ladies' softball team."

It was harder every moment to maintain my composure. But, well, since I was never going to get anywhere with this incompetent bigot who was out of touch with reality, I guessed it was time to give him a reality check.

"Mr. Commander. It is not within the province of a military commander to issue orders to civilians except in cases of martial law, which has not been declared in this state or this nation at this time. It *is* a commanding officer's duty to observe military and patriotic days, and it is a commander's duty to support and protect those in his command. Since I own many volumes of the rule books, I shall be pleased to point out to you chapter and paragraph of each of the laws of the United States military you are breaking."

I walked out of his office disgusted with him and his Middle Ages chauvinism, his bigotry, stupidity, and his flaunting, totally incompetent brand of military leadership. Trying to hold a rational discussion about human problems with this fool was useless and futile.

In the evening Tim came by the apartment to ask about the meeting. I told him.

"The commander is a jerk. He has intimidated his entire command, and nobody would file a complaint against him. I have to tell you, Tim: As Tina's line officer supervisor, I will do all I can to protect her, but the top-gun is *the* commander, and I predict our esteemed SC will make her life miserable."

I nodded.

"He knows he fucked up on all the things you put him on the carpet about. Nobody else ever blew the whistle on him. We underlings who have careers to think about can't. And I suspect he knows in his guts you'd keep whistling all the way to the Pentagon. You are right, you know what you're talking about, and you have that man worried.

"Tim, I refuse to accept that no one has the guts to stand up to this sorry excuse of a man and this disgrace to the military."

"Chuck," Tim said sorrowfully, "the Coast Guard is just a small organization and vendettas are common."

Tim was right. The Station Commander rode her until she blistered. Gave her hell about everything. She in turn took it out on me. She made me the heavy for what happened at the ball game.

Okay, Coast Guard. Take your "Be involved in your station and support its activities" and cram it up your ass. No more "involvement" from this soldier.

A week or two later I was in the club BSing it up with Roger when several of the softball gals came in after practice.
Every last one of them thanked me, one by one, for speaking up for them. Here at the station, the grapevine never sleeps nor slumbers, and they had heard about my confrontation with the SC. They thanked me for that, too.

"I can't believe Tina was so pissed off when you went to bat for us," a shortstop said. "She ought to be proud to have the only husband around here who will speak up for his wife. Husband, hell, you're the only *man* on this whole station."

Said another, "Not a one of our husbands came to our aid, and we are wounded and hurt."

Their thanks boosted my ego a little bit, but I knew that nothing would be done. But I had been ordered to disinvolve myself and I had retreated into the distance. Except for the guys at the VVA chapter and Andrea, I was very alone.

27

In a letter dated June, 1988 the VA Regional Office in Newark acknowledged that I filed a Notice of Disagreement in reference to my claim. (I'd like to think the White House went to bat for me.) The letter of acknowledgment included all the documentation I needed to take my case to the Board of Veterans Appeal in Washington, D.C.

I must reply within sixty days or "We will assume you do not wish to complete your appeal and we will close our record. If you require more time please let us know within 60 days."

The Board of Appeals of the Veterans Administration (BVA) is the highest level of adjudication to which a veteran may carry his case. It is still within the VA, but at least I would be allowed to present my case in person. I would be able to answer questions and offer explanations. The board had to listen.

At no time thus far was I allowed to present my case — other than the fouled-up papers the VA composed, misplaced, lost, and failed to forward. Neither was I ever notified when an appeal was about to be heard. At no point in the appeals process are veterans allowed to present their case in person to decision makers. The veteran knows nothing of any hearing until he gets his after-the-fact copy of the results.

If the appeals board allowed vets to appear in person sooner along in the process, it would lessen the BVA's overload. Decisions would be handed down sooner. If the service rep who is the vet's spokesman can not explain details and finite points that make or break cases then who is left to do it? The veteran's presence would sure as hell eliminate the adjudicator from basing decisions on incomplete or erroneous information.

As before, the VA was *assuming* I had received the letter, and if I had not, as has happened in the past, my case is closed and tossed in File 13. I guess it would bankrupt the system for the VA to send these life-and-death documents certified, return receipt.

First I studied the documents — more forms to fill out, what can I say? — to determine what I needed to gather. Fortunately I had sixty days, because I needed some additional information from Washington state. I sent the request out the same day.

Deep down I really never expected anything to come of my letter to President Reagan. Then I received a letter from Newark.

Veterans Administration

Newark Regional Office

July 19, 1988

Your letter to the President has been referred to this office since your records are located here.

The evidence shows that you filed a Notice of Disagreement with the disallowance of your claim for an earlier effective date for your service-connected Crohn's Disease. You were furnished a Statement of the Case which outlined the laws and regulations and reasons of our denial of your claim for an earlier effective date. As noted in our letter of June 23, 1988, no action will be taken pending receipt of your substantive appeal.

We are in receipt of additional evidence concerning your pending claim for service connection for post traumatic stress disorder. This information will receive our careful and sympathetic consideration and you will be separately advised of the decision.

Sincerely yours,

Director

Naturally I called Stumpy and Jack. Both reminded me not to get overly excited.

"After seven years of being jerked around, I already had that figured out," I told them. "But if nothing else, the VA has been put on notice that I will go to the highest levels of our government, including the President of this country."

Then I reminded them, "This isn't just for me alone. If I can hang in there and give the bastards a good fight and eventually win, it may give others the incentive to take up the fight for their own rights and entitlements."

"We're here to help you in any way we can," Stumpy said, speaking for all the guys at the chapter.

From my doctor in Washington I received a letter stating the history of my Crohn's disease.

Despite the moves in my favor, though, I was still pretty wary. I trusted the VA about as far as I could throw the building that housed their offices.

Late one afternoon in July Tim came by to have a drink. And to talk.

"Chuck. You beating your wife?"

Two things I appreciated about Tim.

He came right to the point.

He had the sense to get the other side of a story before jumping to any conclusions.

Tim explained. "It's common knowledge around the station that Tina often doesn't bother to come home at night. It's pretty obvious she spends all her off-duty time with the guys, even goes out on what I'd have to call dates. Well, Chuck, she told her pals she doesn't come home because she's scared to. Said you've beaten her."

"Tim, the last time I hit a female was when some girl stole my marbles in grade school. My old man beat the hell out of me for that and I have never raised a hand to any girl since."

Tim said, "When I said I didn't believe her, she showed me bruises on her ribs and hips. Get this — she actually dropped her Victoria's Secrets to show me where you supposedly hit her."

I got up and poured more coffee, mostly to hide my rage.

"Uh ... Chuck. You know I don't buy her story."

"Your group's been out on maneuvers pretty regularly lately, Tim, right?"

Nod.

"Water's been pretty choppy, hasn't it?"

Nod.

"Would these bruises be in the same places she'd get bumped around on a wave-tossed boat?"

Tim nodded again and his eyes showed he understood and there was pain in the understanding.

"Tim, if I got mad enough to leave a bruise I sure as hell wouldn't hit her hips and ribs. I'd beat her face in."

The wife-beating gossip spread like wildfire throughout the station. No one on the command staff, nor anyone else except Tim, saw the need to investigate these allegations. That Tina was allowed to stay in the barracks meant the station command gave her permission to do so, since she had her own housing.

It seemed strange that no one caught the big fallacy in Tina's story. If she never came home, just when and where did these alleged beatings take place?

I talked to a counselor at the local army post and made arrangements for both of us to enter counseling. I would see my PTSD counselor and Tina would go to the one at Family Services. We would undergo separate counseling until we both felt we could participate in joint sessions. To my surprise, Tina accepted.

28

On August first I received the paperwork to initiate my appeal to the Board of Appeals in Washington, D.C. First I composed a cover letter to state exactly what I wanted accomplished.

1. Current disability rating for Crohn's disease made retroactive to January, 1981.

2. Disability rating for Crohn's due to increased problems I was having.

3. Seek 100% rating, based on unemployability because of my medical situation. This is a legitimate rating for veterans who otherwise do not meet requirements for a 100% rating for any single condition, but can't obtain work due to their collective disabilities.

4. Health insurance for myself and my family.

I also requested other entitlements important to my survival. Essentially, what I was asking for was the ability to get by in everyday life with a little dignity, and to be able to keep the bill collectors away.

For the thousandth time I looked to the guys at the VVA chapter for encouragement, advice, and assistance. Jack, a member who, as he said, "had access to politicians" (I didn't want to know more about *that* one!), came to the house to review my case with me.

Though Jack had helped others having problems with the VA, he said he couldn't believe what was happening in my case.

"Over and over, your claim has been presented properly and completely, with more than enough to grant all the entitlements you've requested," he said.

"What we need to do now," Jack said, "is to sort out the baseless assumptions and bad decisions the VA made in the past. The first thing I need to do is clarify all the errors made in the past decisions. Then the VA can get on with the real issues."

Jack asked my permission to show a copy of my claim to the United States senator from New Jersey. "Let's put some political heat on the VA," he said, and I cheerfully agreed.

"A legislator seriously interested in veterans' issues could have a field day with my file," I chortled. "Ammunition from hell."

"Okay, Chuck. Prepare yourself to be contacted by the senator's office." Jack was obviously about to have some fun making big waves, because he left with lips upturned and eyes a-sparkle.

Finally, I felt I was really making inroads with the VA. Now I was more antsy than ever about getting a settlement because time was closing in. My marriage was over, and it was critical for me to get myself financially secure enough to take Andrea with me when I left.

It gave me a certain grim satisfaction to picture Tina seriously floundering when she tried to run a household on her own. She had no concept of organizing, of keeping records, or paying bills. Despite her respectable income, she refused to pay any bills or foot any household expenses. Money was to spend on frivolities of instant gratification.

It was almost September — time to get Andrea ready for school. A big second grader now, she was. Fortunately or unfortunately, depending on how you look at it, Andrea hadn't grown much over the summer and last year's school uniforms still fit her. The nuns let us know they didn't want us to get behind in Andrea's tuition as we had done last year.

"I'm going to need your help with the finances," I told Tina. "We can't afford to be dipping into Andrea's school money."

"Her tuition and clothes are your responsibility, Chuck. Those are household expenses and that's your department."

"Tina, you know from experience that my income alone can't cover all the house and family expenses. This is your home and your child, too. You have to kick in and help."

"Can't do. I need my money. You'll just have to watch your budget more closely. Like stop writing letters and buying stamps."

Tina and I were still in counseling. She had her weekly sessions and I went to mine. I couldn't see they were doing her any good; her behavior and our relationship steadily deteriorated. Which was kind of an accomplishment, because when things start out at minus one hundred it's hard to go downhill from there.

By mid-September I was so disappointed and puzzled by her lack of progress that I went to talk to Tina's counselor. "Tell me what I can do to improve things between us," I told him. "I'll meet her ninety-five percent of the way if that's what it takes."

That's when I found out she hadn't been going. She had skipped the last five weeks of sessions.

That very same day Tina breezed in and informed me that her counselor recommended she divorce me *right now.*

"Gee, when did he tell you that?" I said lightly. "This very morning I saw your counselor and he told me he hasn't even seen you for over a month."

She struck with the fury of a typhoon, hurricane, and a woman angered, all rolled up in one. How dare I check up on her? What made me think I had anything to do with her personal business? — as if our marriage is none of *my* business. She went on and on.

This time I sat back while she spewed forth. Made-up accusations and imagined grievances. Her tactic was to redirect her lie with accusations and insults to me, trying to get me to defend myself and get off the subject of the original problem.

This time I knew what she was doing and I wasn't going to let her off the hook. I let her rant and rave until she was finished (or winded), then I returned her to the subject at hand. Divorce.

"See, Tina, if you had been meeting with this counselor all along instead of lying about it, you would know he is adamantly clear that his businesses is to save marriages, not break them up. But he can't do anything for anyone who doesn't show up."

The counselor had hammered it in on me that if I really wanted to work things out I would make sure Tina made all the sessions. Yeah, sure, like I could *make* her do anything.

"Tina, you have got to come out of your fairy tale land and confront real life and the real people in it. You make up lies, then ask inexperienced children who don't know anything to give you advice about problems that don't exist. Then you blunder and mess again and blame it on bad advice. You lie, then you have to tell another lie to protect the first one. Your life is snowballing, Tina, and you're going to get crushed in the avalanche."

Tina coped with the confrontation the only way she knew how. She headed for the club to bitch about me to her stooges. She was going off to get more sympathy for situations that didn't exist, more bad advice about problems she made up, from kids who didn't know anything.

I wanted to hold this marriage together!

Why? Let me count the ways.

Because I didn't want to become another statistic as a Vietnam veteran who has gone through multiple marriages. This is one of our legacies as Nam vets. Multiple marriages. With the highest divorce rate among our contemporaries.

Because marry, divorce, marry, divorce causes problems for our society that are mind boggling. Women on welfare. Children growing up in poverty.

Because the pattern is enduring, the effects long lasting.

Because the physical, social, and psychological problems the man brought home from Vietnam made a generation and a half of women try to be social workers. The man's ladies believe, wrongly, that they can "help," that they can "change" him, but they can't because they cannot begin to comprehend his real problems.

When these well meaning, genuinely loving, caring, compassionate ladies help, they get wrapped up in the uncaring system that really doesn't give a rip about their man. This leads to two problems.

First, the wife is influenced by the mainstream who thinks there is really nothing "wrong" with her man, that the veteran is simply looking for a free ride. Frustrated with her inability to get to him, to help, rehabilitate, and "make a difference," she stops believing he does in fact have problems. As a result, she either gives up on him or she nags him into oblivion.

Second, she constantly gets stonewalled by bureaucratic runarounds, stalls, and denials that the man has a physical, emotional, financial, or employability problem.

In either scenario, it eventually wears down the wife (or more accurately, *all* the man's wives), physically, spiritually, mentally, and emotionally. It destroys the vet, too, and in the process, the family structure and the marriage.

When the marriage implodes, all the legal and societal traditions kick in.

Wives get the children, no matter how unloving, immoral, or abusive they are as mothers. Too often, judges decree that the "psycho vet" is too unfit or unstable to parent, and veterans are ordered to have no contact with their children.

The ex-husband is ordered to pay steep alimony and child support, no matter the wife's work experience and career status, and no matter it was the husband's unemployability that catalyzed the divorce in the first place. It's really difficult to scrape up a thousand dollar a month alimony payment out of a three hundred dollar income. Result: Homelessness, crime, jail.

Many of these men need nothing more than sensible counseling — not the "poor you, you are only a victim" approach, but pragmatic, you-are-in-control skills and awareness counseling — to get their heads screwed back on. And they need some respect and support from the country they served. Not a free handout, but dignity, respect, first-class citizen status, and some training.

Men who have fallen into the abyss must not be brushed off as another bum or deadbeat. Most of these guys need to be told, flat-out and frankly, that they need help; they normally do not look for it themselves. The women involved in these relationships also need counseling.

Much of the Vietnam vets' problems are due to the lack of support they received upon returning home. The failure to address post traumatic stress disorder as a genuine and unimagined disability, and to identify those who need help. Failure of the Veterans Administration to properly meet the needs of the physically and emotionally disabled. Stereotyping the Vitenam vet as something less than a second-class citizen — not of a sufficiently highly placed family to buy a deferrment or too dumb to evade the draft. The anti war movement was, in human and social terms, one of American history's most destructive legacies.

In the anti-Vietnam War movement, the blame and burden were carried by the participants in the trenches who were only following orders set forth by policy makers. It was a debacle conceived, carried out, and supervised by politicians who were sequestered in their elegant offices in our nation's capital.

Politicians who were, by and large, bought by profiteers and goaded on by personal ambitions of status and power.

I have heard leaders in the good old boy organizations, the VFW and the Legion and the DAV, moan and wail and cry and there are lamentations and gnashing of teeth about the decline in membership of their fraternities. "We're dying out," a VFW leader mourned in a speech. "We must get new members." Think about that. To get new members of the Veterans of Foreign Wars, we'd have to have some new foreign wars, now wouldn't we? I hope the veterans' organizations do vanish. Put war out of business. I submit that what the VFW'er was actually grieving was his loss of power. His loss of a job. Like so many jobs, his was created from adversity — war *is* an adversity, you know — and too many adversity-job holders don't want adversities to heal, else they become unemployed.

In the decades since Vietnam, the Love Children, and their New Age liberal successors, it has been rightly said that "people's misery" is America's growth industry. There are more shrinks, social workers, support groups, rehab centers, shelters and safe houses, "victim" advocates, and personal and financial "crisis counselors" than there are teachers. There are untold thousands of for-profit businesses which think up new crises of the human condition, convince people they suffer from it, and charge them to come in and talk about it.

By the same token, one could make a damned good case that the VA's failure to act, serve, and produce creates job security for its employees. If they made cars that didn't wear out, all the mechanics would be out of work; if they discovered a prevention for the common cold all the doctors' offices would be deserted. As long as VA people can mess with (and mess up) veterans and keep them on a string, VA employees have job security.

What makes the VA so insidious is that there is no accountability. If your auto mechanic is inept you take your business elsewhere. If you don't like an elected official you recall, impeach, or vote him out of office. You choose your plumber, your accountant, your brand of cereal. VA employees are not elected and the veteran can not choose his representative nor take his business elsewhere. There is no watchdog agency, nobody adjudicates the adjudicators, and taking your case to a higher level means only that you carry your file folder to another room in the same building. If you can catch anyone when they aren't planning the next party.

29

On the fifteenth of September, 1988 a group of us VVA men car-pooled it down to Washington, D.C. to support House Resolution 639, which was soon to be discussed in the House Committee on Veterans Affairs. If passed, HR 639 would allow the formation of a new federal court to oversee the VA, allow veterans their consititutional right to appeal to a federal court, and address the $10 fee limit for lawyers representing our cases.

We gathered at Stumpy's house and caravanned to D.C. On the ride down we discussed previous testimony to the House Committee.

Over the past twelve years only 12.7 percent of veterans were granted the awards they sought. The number of awards from the Board of Veterans Appeals varied by only 1.3 percent from year to year. In any system which serves clients on a first-come basis, and whose cases are widely and wildly different, the percentage of awards is simply too small and two uniformly consistent over the years to be the result of case-by-case consideration. "In other words," I told my car pool, "this smacks of a quota system."

"Quota?" Jay said. "Sounds more like rationing. Which the VA says it doesn't do. You all know if the VA says it doesn't, it absolutely doesn't, 'cause you gotta believe the VA, right?" Everyone guffawed.

We discussed merit raises and bonuses for VA employees. One of the guys said, "I think every VA clerk is given a bag of money. Whatever he can avoid awarding to veterans, he gets to keep."

Much to our glee, we had obtained a transcript of previous testimony to the Committee. It included a "List of 27 Unfair Practices Used by the VA."

The Veterans Administration (VA) has subjected veterans to unfair practices and procedures for the express purpose of maintaining the integrity of their quota system of dispensing justice. In the process thereof, the VA has adopted **universally creative, deceitful and cunning practices** designed to cause veterans to abandon perfectly valid claims in utter confusion, anguish and frustration and to have been overcome by a deep sense of betrayal. Practices so unfair that in their totality serve to **deny** veterans **a fair and impartial hearing.**

Enumerated below are but 27 of those unfair practices, either engaged in or supported by the VA **in collusion with** the American Legion, VFW, DAV:

1. No right of **Judicial Review** or to have claims litigated in a court of law based upon their individual merits, irrespective of how arbitrary or capricious VA decisions may be.

2. No right to **retain an attorney** in VA claim actions. Attorneys who accept more than ten dollars are subject to **imprisonment for two years** at hard labor and a five hundred dollar fine. Under such circumstances, no attorney will pick up the phone today, much less represent veterans for ten dollars.

3. No right of **subpoena**.

4. No right of **cross examination**.

5. No right of **independent appeal**.

5. No right of **independent medical testimony** to resolve differences in medical opinion.

7. No right to compel VA to **address or confront evidence**.

8. No right to copies of VA **regulations** utilized against them.

9. No right to **discuss case** with the VA.

10. No right to obtain **answers to questions** whether written or oral.

11. No right to **investigate** or explore reasons for **missing files** or records which could prove beneficial to claimant.

12. No right to **personal hearings**, despite regulations to the contrary.

13. Claims are often denied for failure of veterans to answer **correspondence which was never sent**.

14. **Responses** are often vague, obtuse, and couched in bureaucratic language **devoid of meaning**.

15. **Questions** which are deemed repetitive are **not answered**, despite the fact that no answers were forthcoming previously.

17. Little or **no assistance in developing claims** is provided veterans despite voluminous Congressional testimony to the contrary.

18. VA's version re: recitation of the facts is **always accepted**, contrary to any evidence introduced by the veteran contradicting (the VA's) alleged facts.

19. In a rush to judgment, VA often **renders decisions** without benefit of the service or medical records and **without any facts** bearing upon the merits of the claim.

20. **Hearings** are often held without notification of the veteran. A check mark denoting some unnamed Veterans Service Officer's presence is the only indication that some representation was afforded the veteran. Often the hearing record fails to disclose whether the alleged representative said or did anything in the veteran's behalf.

21. After hearings are conducted, **decisions** are often rendered **by personnel not present** at the hearing.

22. VA **employs 800 attorneys** to represent the government's interest but the **veteran is not entitled** to any meaningful **legal representation**.

23. VA rules, regulations and operating procedures are **complex**, confusing, contradictory, voluminous and subject to **constant change**.

24. On occasion, unqualified or **incompetent doctors** are hired and placed into sensitive positions requiring them to render medical judgments and the speed of one or two per minute. Often such medical personnel are unable to secure employment elsewhere and consequently, **easily intimidated** into accepting VA requirements for "agency favored medical opinions."

25. Veterans are not granted the **benefit of the doubt** despite rules, regulations, and sworn testimony to the contrary. Many times, there isn't a doubt, but still claims are denied.

26. In a desire to deny claims, the VA often **invents medical theories** out of whole cloth. Such theories usually **defy** past or current **medical wisdom** or any likely thereafter.

27. Claims before the Board of Veterans Appeals are **successful in one of eight claims.** The allowance percentage rate of 12.7% **never seems to vary** much over the years, no matter how many claims there are — usually 30,000 - 40,000 per year. The percentages which are in such close proximity year after year strongly suggest the **imposition of a quota system** of dispensing justice.

Moreover, it **does not seem to matter** who represents a veteran — whether the American Red Cross, the American Legion, VFW, DAV, self, attorney (pro bono) — the failure rate of 87% remains constant.

According to further testimony, VA adjudicators were paid bonuses for clearing the records of "X" number of cases in "Y" period of time, leaving the "Z" veteran screwed royally. To qualify for these bonuses, an adjudicator must complete forty cases in a week.

Figure it out by simple arithmetic: Forty cases a week means all the medical evidence, legal information, case history, plus all the specific details are carefully examined, studied, checked, confirmed, analyzed, and evaluated; then given thorough, thoughtful, careful, compassionate consideration and a fair and honest adjudication rendered — at the rate of one case per hour. Ha! Then, factor in coffee breaks, attending to personal matters such as party planning, and other distractions ... and in truth, some of the cases are in front of the adjudicator for only a few minutes.

Further testimony revealed that in some cases, medical claims were *denied* at the rate of one or two per minute. Some VA employees processed a hundred or more claims in a week. Now is that thoughtful, considered, serious decision making or what?

Given this, it is logical that an employee interested in making good money could arbitrarily decide to deny, say, the first forty-five claims to hit his desk today and he's in for the bonus. The employee could approve a claim with an equally fast stroke of the pen, except that writing a letter notifying the veteran of his claim approval and award takes extra time; so denying the claim is indeed the fastest way of clearing the books. So what if he is fucking over a veteran who's in a desperate situation.

By testimony to the House Committee, the VA can staff over 800 lawyers to represent them, but a veteran can not enlist an attorney unless it is pro bono. The laywer who charges a veteran more than the allowable ten bucks faces two years in jail and a fine of $500. Congress has not seen fit to update that statute from the Civil War era.

The VA says it wishes to avoid the adversarial approach. By the VA's gifted-mind logic, if the veteran is represented by counsel it's adversarial; if the only attorney is the VA's lawyer, well then there's no one for the attorney to argue with, so it isn't adversarial.

A VA whistle blower, through anonymous letters to lawyers representing some California veterans, stated some methods the VA uses to frustrate and intimindate veterans into abandoning perfectly legal, legitimate, valid claims. Quoting the committee record:

> a) **USING DECEPTION** to deny hearings at crucial times and sensitive stages of the adjudication process. Perpetrators (thereafter are) rewarded with exceptional evaluations, promotions and merit bonuses.

b) **RUBBER STAMPING** of medical rating decisions at the speed of one to two per minute.

c) **DENYING CLAIMS** for failure of veterans to respond to correspondence (which the VA) never sent.

d) **FRAUDULENTLY ENHANCING** productivity performance records to achieve merit bonuses and to promote empire building schemes.

THESE TACTICS were creatively and cunningly developed over a great number of years for purposes of safeguarding the VA's quota system of non-adversarial injustice.

The same informer also reported that, at the request of attorneys representing California veterans, the court ordered the VA to hand over documents and other evidence. The VA destroyed it.

Some of the VA's own employees testified. According to the Committee records:

a) **VETERANS** are not being treated fairly in accordance with the VA's own rules.

b) **CLAIMS** are being prematurely denied without advising veterans of their right to appeal.

c) **CLAIMS** are being denied for failure to provide (information which the VA demands but which is unnecessary to the case).

d) **VETERANS** are often required to furnish service records which are the responsibility of the VA.

e) **VETERANS** are requested to provide income statements although this information was irrelevant to the claim.

f) **VETERANS** who supply income statements (which the VA is not supposed to use in the first place) can be denied their claims (when a VA clerk decides the veteran has enough income without VA supplementation), although income is (legally) irrelevant to the claim.

These same employees told of a veteran who lost both legs in combat in Korea, and, as of 1988, thirty-two years later, had never received any disability benefits. The VA turned down the vet's claim because he "failed" to supply information which he was not even obligated to provide; that information was the VA's job.

Our trip to Washington was for naught. On our arrival we discovered that HR 639 had been sacked. The chairman of the committee invented a new one, a "compromise" he felt would be better. In legislative lingo, "compromise" means watered-down. The compromise to HR 639 was worse than water; it took away some of the few rights we did have.

The only votes against the compromise bill were cast by two California representatives. Once again America's veterans were betrayed. I recalled a passage from the hearings: "Youngsters and their families are not advised prior to entering the United States Armed Forces that injury sustained therein will deny them access to the system of justice they sought to defend."

If murderers and traitors must be read their constitutional rights, then why not youngsters and their families?

After the vote was cast, we vets raised holy hell in the hallowed halls. Media guys were all over us.

A smiling newsie thrust a mike in my face and chirped cheerfully, "How do you feel about this resolution defining veterans' rights? Is this a stirring victory for sensible fiscal responsibility?"

Well, you know which direction she's coming from. Pre-spinning the news.

"If you had studied the resolution, studied the compromise, and were familiar with the legislation HR 639 attempted to reform," I said to the newslady, "you would know the so-called compromise which was passed did not, quote *define* any rights at all. It took away the few veterans' rights that were ever enforced. This is just one more double-cross of America's veterans, just another example of this country's strange concept of justice. I can not understand why a group of Congressmen wants so desperately to deny our veterans the right to appear in court."

I looked straight into the red eye of the camera. "If the media is so dedicated to discovering the real news, I suggest you find out about the secret deals made behind closed doors that shut us veterans out."

In the House corridor, I intercepted a Congressman who was not on the committee and who had no way of knowing what had just gone down. Still having the attention of a cadre of reporters, I asked the honorable representative, "Do you feel veterans are second class citizens who do not deserve the constitutional rights of other citizens?"

The honorable rep had no idea what I was referring to nor of the context of this accostment. But the poor guy was cornered and the reporters all waited with pens poised on pads. "Well ..." His eyes darted from reporter to reporter and he cleared his throat. "All American citizens are entitled to equal protection under the Constitution."

Standard Quote Number Three, generic answer, affrmitive noncommitment when ambushed at the pass. That was fair. After all, I had blindsided the poor guy in the presence of the press.

"Well, guys," Stumpy said sadly, "it's clearly obvious that we vets are being out-lobbied by the VA itself."

I nodded. "I'm convinced the VA is scared that its mistreatment of veterans would be publicly exposed if we were permitted to be heard in a court of law. The corrupt management system than stonewalls us would be exposed, and all those bureaucratic carreers could be forfeit.."

"Dream on, Chuck!" Jay laughed bitterly. "The whole shittin' system is so friggin' corrupt there ain't one thing one bureaucrat could do that's bad enough to get him canned."

After our hell raising almost got us escorted off Capitol Hill, we went to lunch. Next stop: The Wall.

30

The Wall!

The living memorial of over ten years of this government's indecisiveness; of its politicians' disgraceful attempts to be military leaders, and military leaders trying to be politicians. Of politicians hamstringing a military and of political gerrymandering while this country's youth bleeds to death in a war they aren't allowed to win.

Living memorial, yes. Because that Wall lives and breathes in the minds and hearts of every veteran who served in that tragic debacle, and of friends and families they too soon left. The cold marble, warm to the touch. That wall is as alive to us Vietnam veterans as any living creature on this earth.

While we were there in that hellhole in Southeast Asia, we never had time to care about each other as we might have, never had to say good-bye to the fallen. We blocked out real feelings to escape the emotional pain. Now we have our Wall, where finally we can express the feelings we couldn't before and make no mistake about it: that wall lives and breathes. I swear it actually responds to everyone who touches it.

Before this day, I had other opportunities to visit this wall. I would not. I know too many names engraved on that black marble. I have had nightmares about coming here.

As we began our walk to the Wall, I was overtaken by a fear like none I have ever experienced. Unable to continue forward, I angled off, giving the Wall a wide berth. Stumpy and Jay stayed with me, explaining they, too, felt fear and guilt at their first trip to the wall.

First I walked around the far side to look at the statue of the three soldiers.

As I looked on them, those three young men came to life. In the eyes of this statue I saw the war once again. The thousand yard stare, the whole tour that was 'Nam. Time stopped and I was back there. To a time of the most intense fear and pride a human being can experience, for himself and for those going through it with him. For an hour I talked in my mind with those three young men.

Finally, walking between Stumpy and Jay, I slowly went to the Wall.

My eyes began burning.

Surely this is a living, sentient being, for inanimate objects can not so affect a man. As if I were picking up that Wall, carrying it on my back. Embracing all my fifty-eight thousand brothers on it. As we walked the length this tribute to my fallen comrades I acutely realized these brothers of mine will be forever young and never forgotten by those whose lives they touched. Never forgotten except by a government which first denied its young had suffered then denied they had died in vain, then refused to memorialize.

I cried.

As we continued along the wall, scanning the names, I suddenly was looking directly at the name of a buddy, a man who had been a friend since youth. You must understand that this Wall is nothing but a list of over 58,000 names; the odds of spotting a name by chance are truly remote. Yet my friend reached out and grabbed me. I touched his name in the marble and Jay and Stumpy understandingly went ahead.

My fingers traced the engraved letters in my friend's name and I felt surrounded by warmth. At last I was able to say goodbye to an old and trusted friend.

While my hand rested on the marble, I heard words in his voice. "Everything is all right, we are at peace now. Don't let this happen again. Don't let anyone forget what we have done. Help the ones among us who are not back home and hold a place in your heart for us all. Do what it takes to make our efforts worthwhile."

A joke, it's all a god damned joke. A tribute to some magnificent men struck down because of the stupid decisions of our nation's leaders. Voice On My Shoulder wept with me.

I thought of our President's and Congressmen's statements as the dedicated this memorial. That day, our nation's leaders speaking of Vietnam warriors' heroic deeds and dedication; the next day, passing legislation shutting us out from the very rights we so "heroically and dedicatedly" fought to uphold.

The dedication speeches ... to them, the Wall was nothing more than just another whistle stop on the campaign trail. One more place for politicians to wrap themselves in the flag, flanked by a color guard of veterans. Veterans' issues — good politics, but kind of a lot to deal with. Drop 'em as soon as they count the votes and you say *I do so swear.*

I was awash with harsh feelings and emotions, and the tears they brought. "You are better off where you are," I told the names on the Wall. "The hell many of us living are in is worse than the war was."

For the first time in this country's history more men have died by their own hand than were killed in the war they fought in: over one hundred thirty thousand, more than twice the total of names on the wall. Almost every case is directly or indirectly due to an uncaring government and society at large. "Christ," I told the names on the Wall. "We should erect another memorial to the insensitivity and lies of this country's leaders. We can call it the Vietnam Wall of Shame, and on it will be the names of the suicides."

Stumpy and I sat on a bench in the shadow of the Wall and talked about the plight of today's veterans. We talked about what might happen with today's All Volunteer military if the familiar commercials had a subscript: "If you are injured on duty you will forfeit your constitutional right to a lawyer and your right to go to court to claim your rights or redress your grievances."

Nevertheless, despite the rage inside, I came away with a sense of pride and healing.

A few days after the Judicial Review Bill got shot down in committee we found out that maybe some of our hell raising did a little good. Apparently many in Congress heard what happened and forced the committee to change its mind. By legislation passed shortly thereafter, a new Class One Federal Court was to be established to hear vets' claims with the VA. However, the extent of the court's power was not yet known, but it appeared it would have only minimal authority over the VA, not empowered to make award decisions. But it would have the authority to determine if a veteran's rights were violated and it to remand an individual case back to the VA for further consideration. At least it was a starting point, and more than we had so far.

We also heard that restrictions on veterans' rights to attorneys were under revision. Attorneys could be paid a fair fee, though a ceiling was put on those rates so the veteran is still protected from the unscrupulous.

I guess some good was accomplished, after all.

31

At our October VVA Chapter meeting a representative from the VA was our guest speaker. Before the meeting, the members agreed we would let him talk, then give the guys an opportunity to ask their questions. Then this sucker would be all mine.

The rep opened with the standard PR lines. Nothing new, nothing true.

Then it was Q & A time. Some twenty questions were pitched, but he directly answered only a couple. The rest of his responses were tap dances, non-answers, and evasions. He refused to discuss Agent Orange. He avoided the demand for an explanation as to why nearly every veteran gets jerked around. He declined to list the entitlements the VA supposedly offered. He tried to defend illegal actions of the VA. Other answers were pure lies.

Then, my turn.

"Why does the VA not send important documents registered or certified, so the VA has proof the veteran did or did not receive them? Here are some incidents ... " I articulated some examples.

Non-answer response.

"Why does the VA lie to veterans, going out of its way to hide or destroy evidence? Here is an example ..."

Politicked avoidance.

Why is the VA so scared of judicial reviews that it disallows them? When we are in disagreement with a VA action, why must we wait as long as a year for a response?

Creative rephrasing of the question, with response based on creative imagination.

Why doesn't the VA allow open access to CFR Title 38 and permit veterans to look up their own regulations to support their claim — especially when the VA is mandated by law to do so? Why is it that no one lets the veteran see the laws that are supposed to be used? Why are we veterans forced to blindly accept the VA's quotations as the real regulations? In a court of law, everyone is allowed equal access to all evidence, all procedures, and all laws pertaining thereto; why not with the VA?

The only good information coming from the entire evening was that, under the Freedom of Information Act, we can request a complete copy of our VA file. "But most of the information is in VA codes and you wouldn't understand what it meant," the rep bullshitted. "If you do want a copy of your file — which you won't be able to interperet anyway — give me your name and I will have your file sent to you."

He didn't stick around to get any names, though. He was on the highway home, fleeing the troops, before the meeting was even formally adjourned.

On the eleventh of October my DAV "service" rep finally reported for work and was actually there to take my call. He had absolutely no idea what had transpired with my case. Incredulous! A man claims to be representing me, yet he did not recall my name, had no recollection of my case, did not know I was given a physical, and obviously had not done one thing to be of "service" to me since my initial meeting with him in August — when he promised he'd begin serving me immediately.

When I explained the missing documents in my file all he did was "assure" me that "those things happen" and there is very little to be done about it.

"What in the hell are you talking about?" I barked. "These things just ... *happen*? Nothing can be done about it? You mean six years of records just get 'lost' and the Veterans Administration, backed by all the power and resources of the United States Government, can do nothing about it? Are you people making book on how long I will persist?"

Then the old fart boogied through the basic bullshit small talk to divert my hostility and worked on covering his ass. He knew all the doubletalk phrases and tactics. He was part of the good ol' boy network.

These service reps are mostly WW II and Korean veterans. They are great at covering the needs of their contemporaries, but even these people care little about Nam vets. They also have been working inside the VA system for so long they are entrenched good ol' boys. Initially these guys are full of energy and interested in your claim, especially if you are a member of the veterans service organization they represent.

They also serve as quite an effective recruiting system for these organizations. The vet coming in for help feels, or is made to feel, that his claim will get more consideration if he joins the organization the rep is plugging. I feel this recruiting scam should be illegal.

The veteran leaves his interview thinking that by joining he has done the right thing, that his service rep is trustworthy and sincere, that everything is under control. Not realizing that the minute he walks out the door the representative's interest in his case disappears. Based on what other vets have told me and verified by own experience, that service rep may never again even think about the poor sucker's case, let alone *do* anything.

These service reps have the knowledge and the strength of numbers to make the VA an honest, efficient *service* organization. Yet rather than stand up for what is right, they take the easier ride on the gravy train. Undoubtedly these gentlemen all started out with the best of charitable and honest intentions, probably even compassion.

Some of them came to recognize themselves as wielders of power, and power corrupts. All, however, soon realized they had no power, no chance for even tenure (let alone promotion) unless they learned to work within a screwed-up system. It became a matter of "work within our rules or get out." Some of them are basically decent, compassionate human beings who despise the system and despise what they are doing. Yet they refuse to allow their stories to become public.

Two weeks later, October 24, I received another piece of mail on VA stationery. I sighed. More BS, no doubt. More "We have received your request for benefits, you will be contacted in the future." Or worse, "We have received your request ... we are all having a big laugh here ... forget it."

Forget it is right. Why ruin my afternoon reading this piece of drivel. I stuffed the envelope in my back pocket and went over to the Washout Pub and rolled a couple of games of mini-bowl with Roger, then went to pick up Andrea, spend time with her, make dinner, and put in some more Andrea time.

Finally, having run out of things to do, I opened the envelope in my back pocket. The letter it contained was not what I expected; if it were, I'd have opened it hours ago. I most certainly would have shared it with Roger. And Tim. And Stumpy and Jay and the DVA guys.

It was an award letter based on the physical I had last month. Normally it takes several months to get the results of a physical. Perhaps the senator from New Jersey did for a fact carry some clout.

AWARD:

Condition of Digestive System 30%
Residuals of Foot Innury 20%
Sacroiliac Condition 20%
P.T.S.D. 10%

Bilateral H.F. Hearing Loss 0%

Your award has been amended to reflect the abovedisability rating at a combined rating of 60%.

Your new disability award will be $689.00 per montheffective 1 March, 1987.

At last I had made a little progress — but not enough. Instead of being elated I felt like the VA had only thrown me some crumbs. Why was I given "Condition of Digestive System" instead of Chron's Disease? Why was I not getting my rating retroactive to '81? As for the PTSD rating, ten percent seemed small given the report from White City. I immediately thought of my missing records and the absence of the White City evaluation in my files.

The PTSD issue was of little consequence compared to the Crohn's disease. My traumatic stress was not from the war but from the frustration and dealings with the VA itself. Here it is the end of October of '87 and I have been actively pursuing this case since January of '81. Six years and ten months for even the first hint of recognition for the Crohn's. I appreciated the $300 disability increase and the retroactive date, but it still isn't right.

I couldn't understand the total disability rating of 60 percent. Every time I added the numbers, they equalled eighty.

I called my service rep.

The rating, he explained, has nothing to do with any added-up total. "The award is based on the overall effect of the problems on your body parts collectively."

Then he spoon fed me a long equation which I worked out along with him. The end result was something like 58 percent. When the answer is rounded to the nearest ten I ended up with a 60 percent rating. According to their formula, the math worked out. It was the formula itself that didn't make any sense to me.

While I had my service rep's attention I let him know I in tended to file an appeal to the Board of Veterans Appeal in D.C. The Board is the highest level of justice open to a veteran. Remember, veterans don't have the right to be heard in a Federal court.

I appealed the following:

1. The 30 percent "Digestive System" rating should be retroactive to January, 1981, the original filing date for that part of the claim. That I was not given a proper evaluation for the condition in the first place was the VA's failure.

2. I requested a new evaluation of existing evidence and an upgrade of the 30 percent rating. I deserved at least a 60 percent rating; 100 percent would not be out of line given I am unemployable as a direct result of the Crohn's condition.

3. I further requested a total rating of 100% based on the unemployability rule. The rule allows individuals with multiple medical problems to receive full disability when their disabilities prohibit them from obtaining employment.

4. I wanted to be presented with a full and detailed list of all entitlements available, including those the VA had not told me about. I would then decide which entitlements I chose to pursue.

5. I asked VA to assist me in providing health insurance for my family. Such a program (called CHAMP-VA, a version of CHAMPUS) is available, but it is one of those closely guarded secrets the VA hopes vets don't hear about.

My service rep heard me out, then informed me he would commence the Board of Appeals paperwork. "You should receive your copies within a couple of weeks," he said. "Your case will be turned over to a service rep in Washington, D.C., since you requested to have your hearing there."

Oh, peachy-keen and goody! Shuffle you and your papers to someone else, somewhere else. Gives everyone yet one more brand-new opportunity to conveniently lose everything. Again. Not so, Voice On My Shoulder. My homework reveals that the board in D.C. makes all the decisions, no matter what the local people say. I do not intend for my claim to be handled by anyone without decision making power. Having a local board hear my case is like going to court and having one judge hear your case and another judge, who was not party to the hearing, make the decisions based on the transcripts. Trust me on this one, Voice.

The rep continued cheerfully. "Due to the backlog at the Board of Appeals, don't expect a hearing date for nine months, maybe a year."

A year!? Waiting a year for the VA to take the next step was not acceptable. It has been nigh on to seven years already. All right, I shall again call upon the Senator from New Jersey to try to get me an earlier hearing date.

I made it clear to the rep that I wanted to appear in person at my hearing. I also wanted to make certain that all facts and information were available to these gentlemen.

After I got off the phone with the service rep I called the VA to find out when I would receive my check for the back pay and when I would start seeing the raise in my regular monthly check. The answer was what I expected: two weeks to a month.

When Tina came by the house (She didn't "come home" any more; she only "came by." There's a difference.), I told her the news.

"I don't believe it," she said.

I showed her the letter.

"Great." She stuffed some make-up into her going-to-town purse and took off to run around with the guys she worked with.

Shit. Even when I won something, I lost.

"I'm taking the car," Tina said.

"Then you need to pick up Andrea at three o'clock after school, or else get the car back here so I can get her."

Tina gave me a snide look. "I am well aware of what time she is out of school."

I thought about Tina's record for picking up Andrea. Nonexistent.

With some hours to myself I began plannning the Christmas gifts I could now afford for my beautiful daughter. By God, this year she would finally have a bountiful Christmas. Additionally, she wanted a rabbit coat for her First Holy Communion, which would be the third of December. Grandma and Grandpa were getting her communion dress and tiara. I hoped to honor her with a party the afternoon of her Communion Day.

The ringing of the phone sliced through my dreaming.

It was Andrea's school. It was four o'clock and Andrea was still there, and would I please get there as soon as possible. She was being kept at the nunnery until someone claimed her.

Immediately I set out to try to find someone to drive me to the school, or to lend me a car. Everyone I knew was either unavailable or would not let me use their cars.

After six o'clock and three more calls from the nuns, Tina finally showed up. Drunk. Raising hell because Andrea wasn't home. Without acknowledging her presence, I walked past Tina, jumped in the car, and drove to school.

Since I was there anyway, the principal seized the opportunity to mention our being behind in tuition payments. Tina still refused to contribute to the family, not even Andrea's tuition. I told the principal I would be getting a settlement from VA and the tuition would be paid in full the day after I received the money.

While Andrea changed into playclothes I made her a sandwich and told her to take it to the playground. I intended to have a blow-by-blow talk with Andrea's mother while the child was out of earshot.

Perhaps Tina could feel me tuning up, or maybe she knew she had some holy hell coming to her. Whichever, she ducked out. "I have things to do and I don't have time for any discussions," she said defiantly. "I just want you to know I'm going up to New York this weekend and I'm taking Andrea with me. Any running around you need to do, do it before Friday because I'm taking the car."

Then she flounced off to the pub, closing the apartment door with a slam that said, just as clearly as if she voiced it, "Screw you."

I felt an explosion inside me. Who in hell did this bitch think she was? So Andrea and I are a problem for her. A twenty-nine-year-old wife and mother, and nothing matters except partying it up with kids eight, ten years her junior, as if she were pretending to be twenty and single.

Several members of her command had seen her fooling around with the guys she works with. They also knew she neglected her child. In past times, commanders disciplined members of their command for adultry and immoral off-duty conduct. In the "old" Army of my day, Tina's behavior would have earned her a reprimand at least, and under a strict commander, possibly even court martial. Tina's superiors, to their credit, had been keeping her toes in the fire while she was on duty, making her life as miserable as they could get away with. She asked for all the misery she got. Now I realized I was having fun watching Tina cry and bitch about her officers lowering the boom, about (sob) not being treated fairly (boo-hoo).

All my focus now was to keep the VA moving. I had the heat on and momentum was gathering and I couldn't let up. The guys at the VVA chapter kept in constant contact, coaching me through all the stuff I needed to have and do for my upcoming hearing. God bless those guys. They were my strength. They even talked me through my problems with Tina. Jack kept the pressure on the Senator's office, keeping me apprised of what was happening.

In reality not much was happening simply because even a United States Senator has little clout with the VA system. His is just another voice in the crowd as far as the VA is concerned. That agency is untouchable, unaccountable. But Jack and the Senator were at least keeping the heat turned up under the VA: they were being heard, even though they got no response.

At the same time, I had to plan what to do, and how, after I hit the road. It was all over with that bitch of a wife as far as I was concerned. I was only marking time until I could afford to support myself when I did leave. I had to try to put up with her shit long enough to get my case closed with the VA. What I worried about was how Tina's mind games affected Andrea. Otherwise, she could screw all the little bastards at the station. Right into an AIDS epidemic, for all I cared.

32

Just before Tina left for a weekend in New York, my check arrived from the VA. Just over two thousand dollars in back pay. I earmarked the largest chunk of it for Christmas and Andrea's tuition. The rest I set aside for Andrea's First Communion, and for Tim's wedding. I was to be a groomsman, Tina a bridesmaid, and Andrea the flower girl.

The wedding. After finding out how much it was going to cost, I reeled, went numb, and went nuts. Tina reminded me to "put a little extra money aside for the wedding" but she didn't mention that *she* didn't want to foot any of the expenses — not Andrea's gown, not hers, not anything.

The other complication was that Tim's wedding and Andrea's First Communion were both slated for the same day, December 3. Andrea in the morning, Tim in the afternoon. Though he was unaware of the burden this staggering expense was placing on us, Tim, being Catholic himself, did understand the importance of the Communion.

"Chuck," Tim said as we cast our lines one afternoon, "it is a special day for Andrea, maybe so special there shouldn't be other distractions to dilute it. If you want to bow out of the groomsman's job, I'll understand. I'll even figure you have your priorities in the right order."

"Do you want to talk to Tina about it, or do I have to?" I asked. I really hoped Tim would volunteer to be the one, because frankly, Tina liked him better.

"Uh, well ... the two of you talk it over, let me know what you decide."

Jeesh, Lewis, even Tim's scared of wobblin' her boat! Stop it, Voice. Don't start in on me.

Well, Tina decreed that we would attend Andrea's Communion in the morning and then rush to the wedding in the afternoon. Her mom and pop were coming down for the First Communion and they really expected to throw the traditional party for their granddaughter. No such luck because Tim's wedding was to be the season's big social do, very expensive and very all-the-trimmings, and Tina just had to be a part of it, even at her own daughter's expense.

"Of course, *you* can bow out of the wedding party," Tina said sweetly. "Andrea and I are going and —" she put on what she must have supposed was coy, come-hither look "— we'll be the hit of the day."

I didn't even consider that royal plan. If I didn't go, she could stay home, too, and give her daughter the attention she deserved on her special day.

In mid-November the office of the Senator from New Jersey advised me that my hearing date should be "within the next sixty days." I shared the news with the guys at the VVA chapter, but with no one else. It was no longer worth telling Tina anything. None of it was any of her business now.

Thanksgiving arrived and as per normal Tina had to invite her entire clan for dinner at the station. They ate and reveled together and I had my own personal Memorial Day alone.

The week after Thanksgiving I ran out of the medication I took to help relieve the constant pain of Crohn's disease. That Friday we went to New York to help Tina's parents move to their new apartment. As the weekend progressed I became increasingly agitated, freaking out at little things. Andrea asked me a simple little question and I exploded on the poor little girl. I grabbed her by the arm, and why I didn't break it I do not know.

I deteriorated into a total basket case. I was so out of it that I don't remember getting back to the station on Sunday. Obviously Tina did the driving; at least I certainly hope so. Monday I went to the hospital and saw my doctor. I explained the situation as well as I could ... then she chewed out my ass.

She told me I was having withdrawals from the absence of my medication. "Don't you know going cold turkey off your medication can put your body into shock? Or death?"

"Hell, no, I didn't know. It certainly would be appreciated if you would let me know these little things when you prescribe this dope." *For Christ sake! What am I supposed to be, a mind reader?*

"In the event of a medical problem that requires surgery, Chuck, do not go under general anesthesia. That could kill you too."

"Well, thanks to all the medical professionals who never bothered to tell me this before. But I'm glad you let me know about it now, instead of waiting until the day after my next operation."

She gave me a new prescription. Then she assigned me to an At Rest station to be sure I came down safely from my little trip.

"Is there an alternate medication I can use? So I won't have to go through this again?"

"There is," she said, "but for your particular condition it would't be effective at all."

I hit the public library and studied my prescribed medication and its possible side effects. I discovered I had been taking an overdose. For a year and a half I had been taking the prescribed 40 milligrams. It should have been two and a half milligrams. As a side effect, the drug attacks cells in the memory processing center of the brain. No wonder I had been going nuts trying to remember things.

A few other choice side effects include the development of liver disease, kidney disease, pancreatitis, glaucoma, and others.

I already have Crohn's disease and I don't need this other stuff. So, with my doctor's severe disapproval, I took myself off the medication regimen. I told the doc that if she could find something with less severe side effect potential I would consider it, but I did not intend to add more health problems because of medication to reduce a health problem. I will live with, and learn to deal with, the pain.

Naturally Tina used my little withdrawal freak-out episode to beef up her position with her family and to underscore her bogus claims that I was unstable. I guess I did look like the raving lunatic. Tina capitalized on this to tell all her little friends at the Coast Guard station that her hubby was indeed a crazy Vietnam veteran. Her version made no mention of my medical problems, nor of the incompetence of the medical professionals who prescribed an overdose of medications and their negligence in failing to inform me of their dangerous side effects.

The irony of it all was that seven-year-old Andrea understood what happened better than the adults. Tina and her family only saw that I had justified their opinion that I was just another wigged-out vet.

Tina hit me up for almost a thousand dollars for her and Andrea's gowns for Tim's wedding.

I wanted to tell her to go to hell ... but it was only three days before the wedding and at that stage I couldn't leave Tim hanging out in the breeze with a hole in his wedding party. I wanted so badly to back out, but I just couldn't bear to be the one to mess up Tim's plans.

I shouldn't have, but I gave her the money.

With that, my entire two thousand dollar award from the VA was wiped out. Tina had already blown the first half of it on ... a "home entertainment unit," for God's sake. An ostentatious behemoth occupying a whole wall of an apartment she scarcely ever occupied, with shelves and slots for electronic wizardry we didn't own to play music Tina bought for herself but never brought home. She never consulted me about the purchase; she simply took the money from our account the day after I deposited it. I was stunned numb at her unspeakable selfishness, and angry at myself for allowing it. I should have taken her name off our joint account months ago, but I simply had not gotten around to it.

Why did she squander my back pay, and why did I let it happen? Two thousand dollars. The result of seven years of battling with the VA. Gone. Not one cent of it for things we needed. Andrea's tuition was still in arrears and I hadn't a decent suit for job interviews — assuming I would ever have any. We still had overdue bills, no bed, no washer or dryer, and the car urgently needed major work.

On the third of December I awoke wired-up for the crammed-full day ahead.

Tina's mom and pop arrived just past the last possible minute: We were already in the car, ready to go to Andrea's Communion. My girl was a little doll in her white gown and rabbit-fur jacket.

After the service we rushed home, without even taking a decent amount of time to observe our child's solemn rite of passage. We changed, grabbed our stuff, and roared off for the wedding, leaving Mom and Pop alone at the apartment. Strange as it seems, I felt bad about leaving them like that. They came to honor their granddaughter and to throw a party that didn't happen. I wondered if they understood that their daughter put her social life ahead of their grandchild's spiritual well-being.

After the ceremony at the church and the taking of photographs, we were limousined to the reception hall for the partying.

One by one, bride, groom, parents, and attendants were escorted into the hall and introduced. Each walked in, very proper and dignified. Except Tina. When she entered she decided to do some crazy dance step onto the floor. Little Miss Social Standard Of The Coast Guard Station made a total idiotic ass of herself in front of two hundred people. I had not been so mortified in a long time. Derisive titters and embarrassed shuffles rippled through the crowd of onlookers. Poor little Andrea didn't quite understand the ruckus, but she knew something was going wrong.

As the party progressed, Andrea almost stole the show from the bride and groom. She danced with everyone who was willing to be outshone by a midget; and Tim, bless his considerate heart, made it known that Andrea had celebrated her First Communion that morning. That set well with the predominantly Catholic assemblage.

As the evening progressed Tina started warming up to me. In the slow dances she nibbled on my neck and ears. I was thinking I just might lucky after we got home. But I was also prepared not to — I couldn't tell if she was putting on a show for the onlookers, or behaving herself for Tim's sake, or if she really wanted to get cozy when we got home.

Having had my share of drinks, I let my hair down. I danced with every female in the place, including my daughter, who was having the night of her little life. I wasn't doing too badly for a man whose wife claimed he couldn't dance.

It was nearly one o'clock in the morning when the reception was over, the hall cleared, and the last one out turned off the lights. The limo ferried us back to Tim's house, where we changed clothes and claimed our car. I had stopped drinking by eleven, and between that and all the oxygenating activity, I was in good enough shape to drive home. A worn-out Andrea conked out before we were on the roadway.

As soon as we got in the car I found out that Tina had been putting on one of her award-winning acts. She said nothing the entire forty-five minute drive home. She helped Andrea to bed and then took off for the station, where she spent the rest of the night.

Well, I halfway expected that. Our marriage was over. I suppose I'd have been justified if I just packed up and left, but I didn't have the money for that. And as it was, Tina had pretty much left, anyway. This woman was in her own little world and Andrea and I were not part of it.

33

For once the Veterans Administration did what it said it would do: it turned my case over to a representative at VA headquarters in Washington, D.C. And what a jewel she was.

When I called to touch base with her on December 5, 1988, the Monday morning after Tim's wedding, she and I had been talking by letter and telephone for only two months; but in that short time she had accomplished more for me than the whole entire rest of the system had done in nearly seven years.

The lady was the first person who listened to me. The more she became involved in the case, the more she saw how fouled up it was. When she needed documents or information, she contacted me; when she wanted to make a point or a clarification with the higher mucky-mucks, she collared them and made them listen.

She pushed and pursued, trying to resolve part of my claim — especially the retroactive issue — without having it addressed by the Board of Appeals. She expected everyone involved in my case to actually *work* on it, because she wanted the hearing to occur sooner than "in about a year" as the VA projected. She had earned my trust and confidence.

That Monday morning, after she updated me on her progress on my behalf, all I could say was: "Go get 'em, sweetheart!"

The annual Christmas Ball was coming up in a couple of weeks and station personnel were not happy. A planning committee had been appointed, but the commander overruled all their proposals, including the traditional champagne toast. His church prohibited alcohol; in fact he was so Puritan strict it's a wonder he allowed the ball to proceed at all.

Tina went out and spent a fortune on an evening dress — couldn't be seen wearing the knock-out blue she bought last year, you know. I had no idea where she came up with the payola because she had already spent her whole paycheck and all of mine, too, on pretentious, show-offy crap Christmas gifts for all her dear family. (She did save out enough to get Andrea a Little House book and a deck of Old Maid Cards. She made a big show of presenting them, as if they were really big time, big deal Christmas presents.)

Two days before the ball, Tina came by the apartment to report that practically all the Coasties were going to boycott the party. Instead, she was going to go to work as usual. It was no skin off my hide; I had no intention of going to any holiday bash with Tina. The truth: I didn't want to go anyplace with her, ever again.

The day of the ball I ran errands and took care of household business in town. Upon returning home I placed a call to Tina's office just to let her know Andrea and I were home and all was well. The fellow on duty told me she was not in, had not been in, and was not scheduled for duty that night.

Answering a hunch, I looked in the closet. Her new evening dress was gone and so was all her other female fixer upper stuff.

So! Boycott, my ass. Tina was partying, not working. Another round of actressing, another round of lies.

I can see the Washout Pub from the apartment window, and about midnight I saw people thronging to it. I figured they were continuing the party in earnest there.

I awoke Andrea, telling her I was going to the pub for a while and she could call me there if she needed me. Then I walked over to the pub for only one thing: to mess with Tina's evening.

She was at a table, a bunch of young single guys hanging all over her. When I moseyed over and sat down across from her she just about peed her pants.

"What are you doing here?" she hissed. "You weren't invited. You aren't wanted."

"Just a dependent of the station," I drawled, Gary Cooper-like. "Have every right to come in and have a beer or two or three. Might get all the way snockered, for that matter."

All of a sudden her young friends were gone, *poof,* so fast you'd think they had been vaporized.

A couple of Tina's baseball teammates and their husbands joined us. They were still pissed at Tina for the way she handled the harassment situation at the season opener, and the women had it in for her ever since. So they had as much fun as I did watching Tina squirm and steam. She said nothing to nobody! All she did was sit there and suck her wine cooler, looking ...

trapped? defensive? disgusted? ... she was not having a good time yet.

"Gee, I'm surprised you guys didn't go through with the boycott of the ball," I said innocently.

"Boycott?" "What boycott?" "Never heard about any such thing." "You're putting us on, Chuck, right?"

Tina gave me a good Go To Hell look and she wiggled and twiddled her hair. Real agitated. I was about to expose her and she didn't like it.

"Oh. I thought everyone knew about it," I said, faking surprise. I explained what Tina told me about the boycott, and I dramatized and played it up for all I could milk out of it.

My friends were shocked at the lies.

As for me, I was enjoying myself enormously. I took all the more pleasure from the fact that none of her cronies bailed her out; none of them even came over to ask her to dance. Whatever it was they saw in her, it sure wasn't loyal friendship.

I hung around an hour or so and went home. Mission accomplished. I had put a few people on notice that I was aware of what was going on. I had blown the whistle on her lies. I sent the message that I could pop up at any time and monitor her, and I could mess with her plans if I chose to.

Not that I planned to follow my wife around everywhere to keep her in check. I had a daughter to take care of. The Census Bureau wouldn't count us as a single-parent family, but that's what we were and I was it.

I felt pretty good that for once I had managed to fuck up Tina's plans. What I did was pretty petty, but I had issued her a long overdue payback and I enjoyed it.

The first week in January I checked in with my VA rep in Washington. She said she was hot on my claim and asked me to call her back in a week.

The same week the Board of Veterans Appeals notified me that my hearing was to take place on March 28, 1989.

I also received a letter from Ed Stevens of the Disabled American Veterans, who would represent me at the hearing. He even enclosed a map showing how to get to there, which, in my ledger, gave him plus-points for being considerate.

I called Mr. Stevens, partly to acknowledge his letter, mostly just to initiate personal contact. He was waiting for my records, and when he received them he would inform me.

I was amazed to get a hearing so quickly. Wow! March instead of November. I expected my congressman in Washington and the Senator from New Jersey had a hand in it, and I knew my VA rep in D.C. did. In fact, it was obvious to me that this lady with the polite voice and gentle demeanor could really tighten the screws on anyone who didn't feel like putting in a day's work.

In the afternoon I phoned the news to Stumpy, Jay, Jack, and the rest of the guys at the VVA chapter. In the evening I went to the pub and shared it with Roger. Tim showed up and I got to tell it again.

"You told Tina yet?"

"Naahh." *You won't have to tell her, Lewis. With Roger around, everyone will know.*

Let's see ... now it's the second week of January, hearing's in late March: Two and a half months to prepare. I was going to focus on two things: my little girl, and my hearing. No more messing around with Tina and her bullshit; her ticket was now punched to do whatever she wanted. I had no more time or emotion to spend on her.

I went over every document, every piece of paper in my file. Jack and Stumpy conducted mock hearings with me, rehearsing me on every possible question and answer that might come up. They were unmercifully strict in the thoroughness and accuracy they demanded of me, and I was grateful for that. I had to have everything rock-solid to eliminate every possible misinterpretation or misunderstanding. To say it in terms of the cynic, I had to put an iron-and-steel plug in every possible loophole the VA might find or invent in its relentless pursuit of the denial of justice.

In need of assistance on a fine point, I called my rep at the VA in D.C. Since I had dialed her private office phone number, I was surprised when it was the receptionist-operator who answered. I gave her my rep's name and asked if I may be connected, please.

"She isn't available, sir. She is no longer employed by the Veterans Administration."

Boy, that was a disappointment. And unexpected. As caring and meticulous as she was, I'd have thought she'd let me know she was leaving, that she'd have put me in contact with the person who would take over my case.

I asked if I could please speak with someone else. The clerk asked for my name and VA claim number and I gave her the information.

Pause. I assume the clerk was looking for me in her computer. Then: "There is no one available to help," she said.

This didn't make any sense. That was these people's job, to answer our questions. I hung up, waited a few minutes, and tried again. Same response.

Was I being blackballed by this office?

Then the fact of my rep's sudden disappearance registered in my brain.

Did she quit out of sheer frustration? People of integrity don't hold up long when they try to serve others through an agency not attuned to service.

Or was she fired for trying to do her job the way it was supposed to be done? Historically the VA has had problems with employees who take their jobs seriously.

Or did she step on too many higher-ups' toes? Was she blowing whistles? The VA doesn't like employees to create waves or to point out wrongs in the system.

That 20/20 segment flashed through my mind.

That evening I related to Jack and Stumpy this latest episode in The VA Case From Hell. They knew of VA employees who quit because their high moral principles didn't allow them to treat veterans the way the VA wanted them to. They knew others who stuck with the VA, actually helping vets when they got the chance, knowing that if they got caught they could lose their jobs.

I hate to think my rep may have lost her job because of her involvement in my case, but that is what it looked like to me. It also looked like that office had deleted me and my case from its records. It looked to me as if something very wrong and immoral, perhaps even corrupt and illegal, had gone down. Something was quite stinking at the VA.

34

The envelope attached to the coffee pot that morning in February was addressed simply, Charles Lewis.

I opened it and withdrew a paper titled *Legal Separation Order.*

It was a fill-in-the-blanks form that Tina obtained at the post's legal office.

The sorry bitch didn't even have the nerve to give it to me in person.

I called Tina's mom to see what she knew about it. Naturally her mom was stupid about what was happening. I found out later that she knew about it months before. All the crap Tina had been pulling were part of a carefully choreographed program: step one, step two, step three, cha-cha-cha.

I went to Tina's office just before her supper break. I sure didn't like confronting her in the station, but we needed to talk face to face.

Tina said there wasn't much to talk about. "You can stay until your hearing," she decreed. "Then you load up the car with whatever will fit in and you get the hell out of my life."

"What about Andrea?"

"I already have things set up with a sitter to come when I'm on duty."

That's bullshit, Lewis. She doesn't want a little kid to hinder her lifestyle. She's going to give your child away to her parents.

Custody ... I can get custody.

Without a living-standard income? Being unemployable? Face it, Lewis, she's spent seven years setting you up as a wigged-out, freaked-out, dangerous, weirdo wacko. She has all these guys ready to testify that you beat her, remember? She's carefully cultivated the appearance of poor, mistreated wife. Ain't no judge going to give Andrea to you, no matter how unfit a mother Tina is.

Strange how feelings change. I once loved my wife so deeply she was in the marrow of my bones. Now I felt repulsion and despisement — and now that it's openly over, great release. Actually I should have left long ago. More than once I had the urge to load up the car and take Andrea with me back to Seattle. I just didn't have the money.

My options were approximately zero. My income was barely enough to cover the monthly rent let alone the other material things of survival. And if I didn't get a tune-up, tires, and a new battery PDQ, I was going to be wheelless besides. I was effectively being kicked out on the street.

I called my ever present, ever faithful support group: the guys at the VVA chapter. With pain and difficulty, I told them what was happening.

My most urgent concern now was the hearing — and how I was going to get to it. I told the guys that even though Tina, quote, *promised* I could have the car, I didn't trust her for two minutes on it. "Either the damn clunker is going to drop dead by next week, or she'll try to take it," I told them.

My friends assured me they would "work something out" so I could make the hearing. They would also see to it that I got back to Seattle when I pulled out of The Hook.

I felt I was dodging out on the guys, leaving loose ends untied. I was a nominee for First Vice President of the chapter. I was chairman of the chapter's Community Speakers program. I was the contact person for schools and organizations who wisely sought out vets who had been there to tell students the truth about a war which their textbooks quickly dispatched in two paragraphs.

I received a letter from Ed Stevens, my representative from the Disabled American Veterans. To my surprise, it had the basic when-and-where information and a map of the D.C. area — and nothing else. Immediately I called him to make sure Mr. Stevens was entirely familiar with my case. When I told him I would expedite any additional information he needed, he said he had everything he needed to get my claim taken care of.

"All right, then," I said. "But to make doubly sure, let's go over all the issues I want the board to address."

Mr. Stevens assured me he had everything under control and he was prepared to review all the issues at the hearing.

"I think we do need to go over it," I persisted. "I have more medical information that is not yet in my files. Give me your address so I can send it."

"Not necessary to mail it," he persisted back. "I have enough information to represent your case, but you can bring it if you want when you come for the hearing."

Then he asked again, "You are indeed planning to come to Washington to attend the hearing in person?"

"You can bet your sweet ass I'm going to be there. It has taken me nearly eight years now to get in front of a hearing board of any kind and I am not about to miss this." *I'll be there if I have to steal the funds to make the trip or crawl on my hands and knees. I WILL BE THERE!*

The following day I received from the Agent Orange Commission a form to "fill out and return for further processing." It was called the Attending Physicians Statement. Well, I had long ago learned not to take any government form at face value, so I called the Agent Orange Commission for explanation and clarification.

The person I contacted told me that a large number of veterans were being diagnosed with various varieties of inflammatory bowel disease. They occur pretty clockwork-like at ten years after exposure to Agent Orange.

But just like those exposed to nuclear radiation in the post-World War Two era, the government won't acknowledge any connection between exposure and illness. It's pretty common knowledge around the military bases that World War II prisoners of war who were proximal to the nukes dropped in Japan developed radiation-induced cancers and illnesses. Yet the government, through its VA mouthpiece, denies these men their entitlements. The World's Greatest Power is saying, in effect, Yeah, gee, ain't it just the dangest li'l ol' coincidence how all these vets are suffering the same common illnesses; but it jest don't have nothin' to do with their *military service!*

The problem with evaluating Agent Orange and radiation sicknesses is that there are no obvious broken bones, nothing like a missile or bullet injury. Those are easy to diagnose. Diseases, on the other hand, require massive medical testing and evaluation, which the mighty VA claims not to have the time, manpower, budget, or expertise to properly handle. Problems involving diseases are the problems most likely to be denied by the VA because it is easier and faster to blow the veterans off and hope they will go away.

Despite all the scientific evidence and medical research to the contrary, the United States government continues to deny any relationship between military duty and the development of these diseases. With the willing assistance of all the eager young liberals in the press, the public mind has been bent into thinking all the reported symptoms are "hysteria" and "mob psychology," and that those reporting the symptoms are somehow looking for sympathy, victimhood, or a free handout.

Dioxin, the prime ingredient in the compound known as Agent Orange, is one of the most toxic chemicals known to man, says the Environmental Protection Agency. But the U.S. Government, the VA, and the chemical companies that manufactured the stuff deny that Vietnam veterans' exposure to it was harmful. Together, they have even conducted bogus research projects to prove its harmlessness.

If the substance is harmless, then why do the EPA, the Sierra Club and all the environmentalists of any stripe, and the organic food producers prohibit its use on foliage or food crops? If two drops of Dioxin that landed on an apple eight months ago reputedly cause illness tomorrow or cancer in five years, does the government expect us to believe nothing happens to a man caught in the middle of a ton of discharge of the substance?

Based on information from the Agent Orange Commission, I am convinced that my Crohn's is directly related to my exposure to the chemical. On that point, my ace in the hole is that I remained in the military after exposure to the chemical and the disease surfaced well before my discharge. That makes this a service connected illness, and the VA is obligated to address the issue.

Conveniently, the Agent Orange Commission's form asks everything the VA needs to address my claim. The form is completed by the individual's own physician, so the information comes not from a twenty-second glance by a stranger but from a doctor with intimate knowledge of the individual's complete medical history and condition.

I made an immediate appointment with my doctor and asked her to fill out the form as soon as possible. She also made a couple of copies for my own personal records. She jumped right on it, and that very afternoon I had her response to the questions.

I keyed in on some significant answers provided by my doctor. This physician's statement for the Agent Orange Payment Program would give the VA no out for denying my claim.

1a. DIAGNOSIS: Crohn's disease

b. SYMPTOMS: cramping right lower quadrant. pain mucousy stools. and chronic diarrhea with frequency of 15 to 20 times a day.

8. PHYSICAL IMPAIRMENT (as defined by Federal Dictionary of Occupational Titles)

(X) Class 5 — Severe limitation of functional capacity; incapable of minimal (sedentary) activity. (75 - 100%)

10. PROGNOSIS

a. What is the prognosis? Specify a prognosis for each of the various diagnoses listed. Use a separate sheet if necessary.

Variable prognosis. At this time the patient is undergoing a moderate exacerbation of the disease.

b. How long from now do you feel the patient's maximum medical improvement will be reached?

( ) 3 months ( ) 6 months ( ) 1 year ( ) longer
(X) no improvement expected

The questionnaire included a lot of other general questions relating to my general history, but the ones above were the questions the VA should have asked and had answered almost eight damn years ago. This is one of the best documents a veteran can carry into the VA to support his case. Everything is factual, laid out in black and white, and even a moron can understand it, including VA adjudicators.

I showed the completed form to the guys at the VVA chapter. All of them saw it as my ticket to justice.

"I must remember this form so I can advise every veteran that it could be the difference between their getting or not getting their disability award," I told them.

"Okay, Chuck." Jay winked at me and stood up like he was a teacher in front of the fourth grade. "Say the name of the document three times, and tell the class where to get it."

I stood up and recited in capital letters. "ATTENDING PHYSICIANS STATEMENT. The document is Attending Physicians Statement. Contact the agency called AGENT ORANGE COMMISSION and ask for the Attending Physicians Statement."

"Good, Chuck. Now tell us what it's for."

"The Attending Physicians Statement answers and quantifies the history and level of the individual's past medical history. It is factual and valid because the information is based on the expertise of the veteran's personal physician, who is the one most likely to have long-term and intimate knowledge of the veteran's ongoing condition. The answers resolve and solidify any arguments pertaining to a veteran's past history. Of course the VA can ignore the information, but if they do, the veteran's appeal will be based on the record. Eventually the VA will have to address the documentation."

"That's very insightful, Chuck. Anything else?"

"It is important for a veteran to remember this: You can't ever have too much supporting evidence for a claim with the VA. If there is something I have learned so far it that you must have everything — *everything* — documented. Make two, three, or more copies of everything while you're at it. Because two, three, or more doctors, clerks, representatives, VA offices, or sundry government officials will need them, and at least that many will claim they've lost them at some point along away. The VA can't stand it when you come in with piles of documentation because that means they will have to go through the whole stack and that means *someone* will have to *work*. It is doubtful that anyone does read everything; but if it's in writing, the veteran is covered by having it on record. (Like the manila envelope full of important information tucked in the back of my file; nobody read that until I stood over them and made them open it and read it aloud to me. Then they knew I was witness to their having read it, and they couldn't say they never saw it.)"

I sat down, my pop quiz completed. With his index finger, Jay ascribed my grade in the air. I got an A.

I called Ed Stevens to advise him the form was completed. "I'll bring it to the hearing," I said.

"Yes. I was going to tell you to do that, in case you didn't think of it."

In case I didn't think of it?! Right, like I wouldn't think of taking ammo on combat patrol! What intellectual level did the man think he'd been dealing with, anyway? Now I wondered if he had been giving me some kind of dumbed-down treatment.

In addition to putting together an impeccable file of documents and claim information, I managed to talk to a lawyer. Though he couldn't represent me, he gave me some helpful suggestions.

Does it appear that I didn't fully trust my service rep? I didn't. I didn't trust anyone to do what I could do myself. Especially since the national DAV publicly declared Vietnam veterans a bunch of crybabies trying to get everything for nothing. The DAV was against veterans getting the right to carry their claims to Federal court. It was also against increasing the $10 fee limit for lawyers repping Vietnam vets. On the state level, some DAV people supported judicial review and raising attorney fee limits, but when any organization has a national-state-local hierarchy, there is little clout at the state level, even less for local posts.

According to the transcript of a hearing conducted in November, 1987, the Disabled American Veterans representative said:

> "One of the witnesses that will come before you this morning has described the VA as so fundamentally flawed and institutionally corrupt that the only recourse is to allow determination in the Federal Court system.
>
> "We certainly don't agree with that characterization. We don't believe that should be the basis of the subcommittee's consideration and deliberation of the issue. Exaggerated incorrect statements of that sort certainly do not lend themselves to a consensus that [engaging the Federal court] is in the best interest of veterans and their system. ...
>
> "There are problems inherent to the process. They are related to lack of funding, staff, [and] training; managerial problems, dwelling on the end products, quality control, and measurement of productivity. All these things can impact on the way benefits and handled and adversely impact on the entitlements that are given to veterans."

According to the gentleman, I am supposed to matter-of-factly accept that the VA hides documents. I should just let it slide that the VA failed to notify me of a hearing, not be upset that I couldn't attend because they didn't tell me about it. Just a couple of those casual, inconsequential little things one writes off as bad luck. According to the gentlemen, veteran suicides, failed marriages, homelessness, poverty, drugs, crime, and imprisonment are just matters of "Oops. Little run of bad luck, there, fella."

If caring for its veterans is too expensive, then the leaders of this country should quit trying to be the world's policeman.

35

Tina and I went to the legal office and finalized our separation, effective the end of February. She magnanimously allowed me to stay at the apartment until my Board of Veterans Appeals hearing in March. I agreed to move out the day after the hearing.

Over the years a number of vets had told me their second failed marriage hurt worse than the first. Now I, too, have been there, done that. I had been a long-time divorced man before I met Tina; but I wasn't particularly broken up by that divorce because the marriage had been little more than a blip on the screen of my life. Tina, on the other hand, I had loved so deeply she was in the marrow of my bones.

My only misgiving about the separation was the belief that Tina planned to cut me off from contact with Andrea. Truthfully, my wife was very jealous of our father-daughter relationship. But hell, that was Tina's own fault for not taking any time with her daughter.

I organized my belongings, preparing to pack. I would stack everything by the door before I went to Washington. After the hearing, I would return to the apartment and simply load up and leave.

I had enough money for the trip to Washington, D.C., but as the hearing date approached it was clear I hadn't enough money to get to Seattle. I went to the Red Cross and explained my situation. They took all the details pertaining to my claim with the VA and said they would notify me in a few days, after verifying the information I gave them.

On March 13 the Red Cross spokesman informed me they could not help me. If a veteran is involved with the VA, the Red Cross can help him prior to his *initial* decision. Since I had already been handed down the VA's first decision, I was no longer eligible for Red Cross assistance.

"Could I get just a loan to get me home?"

"I am sorry, Mr. Lewis. It is our policy not to become involved with persons having cases before the VA."

"Let me clarify this," I said. "Right now you won't help me lift my bootstraps? But when I'm on the streets I am welcome in one of your soup kitchens?"

The long, devious arm of the VA even reaches into Red Cross policy making. Stunning.

As of this moment, Lewis, we are looking at the prospect of living on the street. And all this is more or less because your beautiful and wholesome wife is the Free Spirit of the Coast Guard. A whore. You, Charles Lewis, upon whose shoulder my voice dwells, have been dealt the ultimate betrayal. My voice has no words for that feeling.

Listen, Voice On My Shoulder. You know I went to Vietnam and deliberately exposed myself to Agent Orange just so I could get this disease and all the other medical problems to screw up my life. Then be accosted by the VA and their horseshit methods. No wonder so many of my brothers go off the deep end and do stupid shit. Oh, Voice, O Voice, this is the most frustrating and senseless circle of fucked up process and conduct I have ever experienced. That goes for both my wife and the Veterans Administration.

One afternoon in early March while I was doing my normal house cleaning I found some papers Tina left on our dresser. I didn't want to toss something important, so I opened them to look. What I saw was such a shock I could scarcely comprehend the words I was trying to read.

Tina had sworn out a warrant asking the cops to physically remove me from our apartment. According to her statement on the warrant, our separation was in effect but she couldn't get me to leave. She swore that she feared for her personal safety, and that I was armed most of the time and was "extremely dangerous."

What a crock! Couldn't this bitch just leave the battle she had already won?

Tim, a friend to the end, came by that evening. He knew about the warrant. Hell, everyone at the station knew about it because

Tina had been showing it around, flaunting it like it was some kind of blue ribbon. Tim, friend to me and somewhat of a Dutch Uncle to Tina, had talked to her and found out she was still onstage, playing her last act of "Pity Me." She got the warrant to invoke the sympathy of her cronies.

"But she's not going to file the papers. You have nothing to worry about, Chuck," Tim assured me.

"Your damn right I have nothing to worry about," I told my wife's line supervisor. "Tina offered to let me stay until my hearing, and by God she's going to honor her word for a change. But hey, my hearing is two days away. Guess she'll just have to tough it out another few hours. Then I'm out of here."

I got up and popped a pair of cold ones and handed one to Tim. Men understand the gesture of a man handing a man a beer, and Tim would know this was my way of telling him how much I valued him as a person, friend, and confidant. We sipped and small-talked, and I told Tim about last weekend's VVA dance.

We were just a bunch of vets and others interested in our issues getting together for a good time. My good ol' friend Stumpy quaffed a couple too many, as he sometimes does to emphasize a point in the debate he is engaged in, he took off his wooden leg and threw it at his worthy opponent.

When he was a Marine, Stumpy got hit in the butt with a ricocheting rocket from a gun ship. A hard assed Marine. Among other things, he lost a lower leg. I didn't know how to act the first time I saw him take his wooden leg off and throw it at someone; but after that I realized it meant that he accepts his situation.

Once Stumpy told me of his stay in the VA hospital, how unclean and understaffed and uncaring it was, and of the carelessness. Several years after his injury he managed to grab a peek at his medical records, and there he saw in writing something he never knew about himself. He was sterile. The VA had never told him. The VA does not allow vets to see their own medical records, and VA doctors don't tell them everything there is to know about themselves, either.

Soon enough Tim said, "Well, buddy, gotta get home and make the new wife happy."

I grinned. "And I gotta leave home to make my old wife happy." We laughed together at the irony.

I was sure this was the last time Tim and I would share a

beer and talk, and I sort of wanted send him off with a hug. Instead, I my valedictory to him was: "I wonder what her life will be like, not having me to blame everything on."

All my belongings were packed, ready to load into the car as soon as I got back from Washington. After my Board of Appeals hearing, I would stay with Stumpy for a couple of days so I that I could be there to vote in the upcoming VVA chapter elections. The extra days would also take me up to another payday. I would need most of my monthly allotment to get some needed work done on the car.

36

At 3:30 in the morning of March 28, 1989 I headed for The Nation's Capital for my appointment with the Board of Veterans Appeals and what I had been thinking of as my meeting with destiny and my future. The first good omen of the day was that I found a parking place that was in the same time zone as my hearing. The second was that my beater of a car got there.

I reported to the front office and introduced myself. The secretary conducted me to a room and went to tell Ed Stevens I was there. I wandered as I waited, looking around the offices.

In one room were two seven-foot-long tables. The tables appeared to hold stacks of trash six feet high. I moseyed over to take a look at the trash and saw that it was . . . VA claim folders.

While I stared at this chaos, some guy came in with a shopping cart filled with more files. He threw them onto the heap.

What in the hell was this squalid mess? There was about a ninety-eight percent chance of papers falling out of file folders, and the odds were even that stuff would be put back in the wrong folder. I thought of the 20/20 segment showing a mess just like this one. "It must have been filmed here," I thought. "There can not be two offices like this."

I thought of a story I heard about a vet who was taken to surgery and the doctors amputated an arm instead of repairing a slipped disk because the doctors wrong papers had gotten into the vet's file folder. "And," I thought, surveying this ground-zero chaos, "a lot of vets are about to get fucked."

At 8:30 Ed Stevens came into the room and we introduced ourselves. I was comfortable with having a full hour and a half to go over my case prior to the hearing.

First Ed brought me coffee. Then he started small-talking

about everything except my case. I let him ramble a few minutes. Then breaking into his weather report, I told him I brought all the documents to support my case, and I wanted to discuss the matter at hand to make sure we were on the same frequency.

"Well, ah ... um. Well, y'know. The only part of the claim the Board is hearing is the retroactive thirty percent issue."

"WHAT IN THE FUCK ARE YOU TALKING ABOUT?" I was speaking in capital letters. "My request for this hearing included several points of contention supported by my senator and resulting from a letter I sent to the President of the United States." I was yelling. "I spend money I don't have to come here for this hearing I promised to attend AND YOU TELL ME YOU AREN'T ADDRESSING MY WHOLE CASE?"

Ed Stevens sat very still and his eyes evaded mine.

"It took me eight fucking years to get to appear personally at my own hearing and THIS IS WHAT I AM SUPPOSED TO ACCEPT?!" I was on the border line of beating the hell out of this jerk.

"Why in hell didn't you say something sooner? Shit, we talked on the phone yesterday. I don't NEED to be here if THAT is all that is going to be addressed, because that part of my claim is self sustaining on its own merit. I came to testify and answer questions, and to stick up for myself. It's God damn sure YOU ain't getting the job done."

Ed Stevens was cowering now, and I enjoyed that.

"I have the distinct feeling that you are really fucking with me here. You assured me everything is under control and that my case looked good. Now you hand me this shit."

All my mind's eye could see was me beating the streets of some city, a derelict with no future and no hope. My veins stood at attention and the muscles of my hands ached to tighten around this bastard's throat. I was as close to killing as I could get without actually doing it. I do not know how I restrained myself, or why. Too many witnesses, I guess: I had the attention of everyone on the premises. Okay, you morons are standing around for a show, I'll give you one. Curtain, Act Two.

"Why can your Appeals Board Of Fine American Justice not address all the issues as prayed for in my request for a hearing? A hearing your board agreed to hold. Does the Board not have enough brain power to think of more than one thing at a time?"

Some onlookers were working their fists and squaring their

jaws. Merry-eyed others were swallowing their lips to keep from guffawing. What I sensed was an intriguing polarization — the shit-slingers in one camp and shitees in another.

"I just want to know why you and your esteemed so-called service agency conned me into believing you and then stabbed me in the back when I did."

Mr. Ed Stevens backed away and made a bunch of phony excuses. I had read the manuals which veterans aren't supposed to know about, I knew the correct rules, the lawful procedures, and the right protocols (most of which the VA routinely ignored), and I knew his excuses were all smoke and mirrors and no substance.

"When I was an infantry instructor, Mr. Stevens, I taught, lived by, and required my men to adhere to a little motto. ***The maximum effective range of an excuse is zero meters.*** Think about nailing that one on your wall."

Somehow I regained a microscopic measure of composure and Stevens produced another cup of coffee. "The hearing will be held as scheduled," Ed Stevens said in that too-too polite tone people use when they are walking on eggs. "Please stay for it."

Stevens said, "So many veterans ask for personal hearings and then fail to appear. A Baltimore man didn't show up, the board didn't appreciate it, and the vet lost his case. But then, the claim had no merit to begin with."

Stevens was trying to show me that our tiff was water under the bridge, so I responded with the same courtesy. "You mean," I said, "if the hearing isn't important enough to the veteran to show up for it, it isn't important enough for the board to seriously address it?" Stevens nodded. "So not being there is tantamount to losing."

"Yes," Stevens said, "or at least it sure reduces your odds of a decision in your favor."

I decided to stay for the hearing. Not because of Stevens's veiled threat, but because I had spent the money and made the trip.

All smiles and platitudes now, Stevens said, "If you win on this issue, you will at least have some working funds to continue your case."

Yeah, get awarded ten dollars so you can spend eleven dollars protesting that you got only ten dollars.

I smiled a little, glad to know that Voice had retained his sense of humor through the shit storm. Ed Stevens must have thought I was smiling in agreement with him, so he gave me a There, There, Little Boy smile back and continued.

"Frankly, Chuck, I am aghast that your case is taking this long, and I'm surprised it even had to be taken to this office. It should have been resolved at the Seattle regional office years ago."

Platitudes, Lewis. Beware.

Then Stevens chewed me out for going to my congressman and senator. "It only slows up the process when we have to pull files to respond to any legislator."

"Gee, it seemed to speed things up by several years when I wrote to the President. The VA responded in a real hurry when Regan instructed it to move on my case."

Stevens ignored that and went on with the lecture. "Besides, you know, the VA has its own rules and policies and it doesn't have to answer to any legislator, anyway. So in the future," he flashed the kindergarten-teacher smile again, "don't waste your time contacting your congressman."

What a crock! Boy, it's heaped deep in this office. The real reason the VA doesn't want vets to talk to legislators is because the VA doesn't want legislators to step into the VA's comfortable little feudal estate.

At ten o'clock Ed Stevens escorted me to the hearing room. I conducted myself as if I were cooled down but in reality I still seethed. We entered the room first, followed by members of the Appeals Board: a physician, an attorney, and the board chairman, who represented the adjudication division. I took the oath, promising to tell the truth. How ironic, the VA asking for an oath of honesty.

The opening statement came from Stevens, who quoted a list of regulations that were incomprehensible to me. It was such gibberish it was as if he spoke in a secret code.

Then I was "offered the opportunity" to explain my points of contention, and document why I deserved the retroactive entitlement. I summarized the history of my case, the whole sorry story.

Most of the remainder of the hearing was questions and answers to clarify the facts. The questions they asked and the answers I prepared were the ones Stumpy and Jay had so carefully coached me on.

The board members asked in several different ways about

the bogus address the VA used in 1981. The doctor grilled me about the history of my Crohn's disease, which I had explained to them once but feigned patience as I repeated the details. I told the gentlemen I had additional supporting medical records which I wanted them to review. They said it wasn't necessary because they already had enough relevant data.

Preparing to adjourn the session, the chairman asked if I had any other comments. That was my opening.

I called the group on the carpet for leading me to believe that my entire case would be heard, then dealing only with the retroactive issue. I drew them a picture of my financial status, emphasizing that the Veterans Administration was essentially responsible for my source of survival. I told them of having been kicked out on the street and made clear that the basic reason for it was the VA's failure to act on my claim years ago.

I left no doubt in those people's minds that I was very unhappy with them.

As I spoke Ed slowly shrank down in his chair. From what he said earlier and from his demeanor now, I figured out that I was speaking of things he did not want talked about. Somehow it felt as if the board members knew nothing of the other issues I wanted discussed and resolved. But then, they are good actors. I didn't know who was responsible for deleting issues I wanted addressed, but I let them know it had happened and I was not happy about it.

After adjournment, each board member graciously shook my hand, and all apologized that my case had been hanging so long.

The chairman told me I should get an answer in 90 to 180 days. I think that's far too inexcusably long, but I made no comment. He offered to give me a copy of the tape recording of the proceedings. I accepted and went with the clerk to get my copy made.

With the tape in hand, I left the building. I had to get away from *Mister* Stevens as soon as possible, because I still had the urge to do him in. Ed Stevens and all his phony concern could cook in the fiery furnace for all I cared.

As I drove back to New Jersey I mentally reviewed the morning. The hearing itself wasn't as bad as I feared. I felt confident of victory in the retroactive issue; and if I did, it would help my financial state until I could get the rest of my claim addressed. I knew that would take at least another year.

I tried to play the tape to see if I did things right. But it was a poor copy, most of it garbled and incomprehensible. I made a mental note to request a written transcript.

Stumpy and his wife operated a stable on their farm about a half hour from Sandy Hook, where they rented stable and pasture space to local horse owners. My route took me right past the place, so I stopped. Stumpy and I had some coffee and discussed the hearing.

"I'm impressed with the way the board members conducted the hearing," I told my friend. "I think I made an excellent case, and the board was receptive."

"Don't get overconfident," he cautioned. "Don't expect anything from the VA until you actually have it in your hand."

As for Ed Stevens and his watering down of my issues, Stumpy was infuriated but not at all surprised. He had nothing good to say about the DAV. That organization had in the past publicly stated they regarded Vietnam veterans as nothing more than a bunch of crybabies trying to get something for nothing.

"Be sure you get yourself a new rep as soon as you get to Seattle," he admonished.

The Vietnam Veterans of America was soon to start a service rep training program, and Stumpy was to be one of the first in the program. I was glad that we as an organization were finally getting around to getting our own service representatives, to be trained by our own legal staff. Stumpy would make one hell of a rep. He and the other guys tried to encourage me to enter the program, too, but I was too hostile toward the VA and too cynical to deal with such a corrupt system.

I was tapped out with money so I had to borrow a couple of quarters from Stumpy to pay the tolls on the rest of the drive home. Then we so-longed and I of course promised I'd be back the next day.

I arrived at the apartment — tomorrow morning it would be my *former* apartment — and sorrowfully began my last evening with Andrea.

After Andrea was asleep I loaded the car, ready to be on the road as early as possible. Tina would be off duty in the morning, and she surely would be there bright and early to make sure I was on my way out.

I went into Andrea's room and I just sat and looked upon my beautiful daughter. I knew it would be a long time before I saw her again.

Bitterly, I foresaw Andrea's future. A beautiful, bright, vivacious child whose mother only saw her as a financial drain and an impediment to her social life. Tina would simply hand Andrea off, most likely to her parents. That meant being housebound in a one-bedroom apartment in Bronx, where it is unsafe for a child to play outside or go places with friends or have visitors. Grandma and Grandpa were too ignorant to help with schoolwork and extracurricular activities and too old to understand a little child. That was what was in store for Andrea.

In fairness to Tina, her work schedule was not particularly conducive to caring for a child, although it certainly could be worked out if she were willing to dump her self-proclaimed role of Station Socialite. Tina had to serve her Coast Guard hitch; she had an enlistment contract that forced her to fulfill an obligation. This will be the first time she ever saw anything through. She never completed a single college course. She never stayed with any job for more than a month.

Tina was there in the morning, just as I predicted, and woke me up and told me to hit the road, just as I expected.

I went to my daughter's room and held her and assured her that I would always be her daddy and I would always love her. "As soon as I get an address I'll write to you, and you can write to me whenever you want." She nodded wordlessly. "You continue to do well in school, honey — " I held her tighter and kissed her hair " — and be brave about all this."

I left her room and went into the kitchen and grabbed my thermos of coffee. Then I went to the car and drove off.

The last thing I saw was my daughter standing at the door crying.

37

Spring was stirring that morning in late March, and Stumpy was out in it, doing some work on the stables. I jumped in and gave him a hand. As I worked, I began the process of mentally regrouping. I had to put my life back together, and I had to use a different set of pieces to do it.

My car needed a tune-up and break work, and new tires. That was going to be a burdensome expense: buying tires without any money is a real treat. I ended up spending nearly my whole paycheck on the car, even though I did most of the work myself.

Stumpy and I worked on VVA chapter business. As outgoing president, he wanted all the loose ends tied up in a tidy package to hand to the new president right after the chapter election.

On April fifth, I attended my last meeting at the Vietnam Veterans of America chapter. We held our elections and conducted our normal business. Then Stumpy and Jay announced that this was my last meeting, that I was moving back to Washington state. Through the grapevine, everyone there knew about my whole situation, so the announcement was no news flash; it was a diplomatic way of putting it out in the open. It was Stumpy's way of saying We know; we understand; we care.

Then Stumpy passed the hat.

Stumpy poured the contents of the hat into a large padded envelope and presented it with a hug and all the guys and gals clapped. After that we all went downstairs to the bar, had a drink, and I said my good-byes.

When we got back to Stumpy's house I counted the money. Three hundred and eighty dollars! From only thirty people. I was touched and moved.

I will go a long time before I ever find the comradeship and caring this VVA chapter offered. These were men and women who truly cared about each other, who took pride in being there and helping out. Never have I been as closely bonded as with them.

Daybreak. April 3, 1989. I pointed the car toward the west and put the pedal down.

There was comfort in the going. I would no longer have to put up with Tina's lies and cheating and extravagance and her general shit.

There was loss in the leaving. I was losing my child. I was parting from the best group of guys I have ever known.

The VVA group were the only people I could relate to. If you have never been in combat you simply can not relate to someone who has. I am alive and starting a new life because those people cared enough to help me when I needed it the most, emotionally and physically.

I faced the direction of the sunset and drove and drove. I stopped only for fuel and food, and to take little cat naps in Interstate rest areas.

Just west of Salt Lake City, my car's water pump broke. Overheated and dry and stranded in the middle of Great Salt Lake Desert. I sent out an SOS via CB radio. No response. A couple of Utah State Troopers drove right by without stopping. They didn't even slow down to see if I needed help — as if my frenzied hailing were not a clue that I did.

I looked at the options and had to turn each down.

Water bottles: Fell over in the trunk and leaked out. Amazing, considering everything was so tightly packed.

Find stream or pond: In the middle of Nowhere Desert?

Pee into the radiator: Interesting picture, but no piss in bladder. Bladder didn't hold radiator full, either.

There was only one viable alternative, and it was a very very last resort. But I had come to the last resort.

I opened the trunk and took out my booze. Into my empty radiator I poured:

[A] a half gallon of White Label Scotch (a gift from Roger The Bartender, he probably embezzled it);

[B] two fifths of Glenlivet Scotch ($42 a fifth, one from VVA, one from some of the softball gals);

[C] a bottle of really good Irish whisky (from Tim);

[D] a fifth of bourbon (cheap brand, self purchased).

God, did I cry over such carnage of good liquor.

Driving westward, I found a little stream just off the Interstate. Using a tee shirt as a filter, I filled my water jugs and topped off the radiator.

About sixty miles later was a service area. Fortunately the mechanic had a water pump for my make and model. Unfortunately he wanted eighty bucks for the pump and another hundred for installation. I told Mister Rip-Off Mechanic to go screw himself, filled my water jugs, and continued driving west.

I found the car went precisely one hundred miles before overheating. So I got into a rhythm: drive my hundred miles, pull over, let the car cool off, refill the radiator, and drive the next hundred miles. That was my routine for the last five hundred miles into Klamath Falls — back to K-Falls.

From New Jersey to southern Oregon in 71 hours. Man, talk about tired butt and bleary eyes.

I contacted Craig, my friend and classmate at Oregon Institute of Technology. For three days I shot the breeze, slept, laughed, got reacquainted with friends, slept, drank cheap beer, and caught up on some sleep.

For the first time in ages, I got to go out and have some fun without being stalked by the specter of Tina's anger, hostility, and infidelities. It was terrific. I was living again, alive for the first time in years. Craig and the rest of the guys weren't surprised about the Tina situation; they had been conspirators in the anniversary debacle, a scene they well remembered.

My time with Stumpy, my driving time of solitude, my time with Craig and friends — *friends*: I had already begun to heal. But now it was time to head north, where I could stay with my mom and dad for a while. It was the only place I could go and get some help until I got the results of the Board of Veterans Appeals hearing.

I hit the road for the final drive home and back into the world of sanity. When I pulled up to my folks' apartment, I still I had three whole dollars in my wallet. Thank you, Stumpy and Friends.

PART THREE

38

For the first time in ages I was at peace. No longer need I be on constant guard from another one of Tina's emotional attacks. The guilt of a failed marriage was not mine; I did try and I tried really hard. Now I am home where I am accepted and I do not have to live with the embarrassment of her conduct — or the fear of it.

But: My parents lived in public housing. By regulation I could stay with them for only two weeks. On $700 a month from the VA, it would take me a long time to save enough to get my own apartment.

After explaining my situation to the Housing Authority, though, I was added to my parents' lease. Of course, the rent went up because my money constituted additional household income, but that was fair; I contributed the increment. Due to my low income and the fact that I was a disabled veteran, I qualified for my own housing, and I gladly accepted the opportunity to be placed on a waiting list for my own apartment. I say it was an opportunity because I was a low-priority placement. Everyone including illegal aliens was of higher priority than I as a single veteran — or a single man at all, for that matter. I knew I could remain on the waiting list for years.

I got back in touch with Ted and it was of those little full circles of life. My former classmate, fellow employee, my business partner-to be ... now he, too, was divorced; and now we went fishing together and black-powder target shooting again, just as we had done before. Now he was back in school, finishing up the drafting degree which we began together, and I would return to school, too, this coming term.

Just as I was sure she would, Tina gave her parents custody of Andrea. Complete legal guardianship. Though I called my child repeatedly, her grandparents did not allow her to talk with me except for an occasional three minutes. Once, at summer's end, Andrea called me from a friend's house. It was then she told me she never received a single one of the weekly letters I wrote her. I hadn't received any of the letters and pictures she gave Grandma to mail to me, either.

At Green River Community College — another homecoming, another circle — I enrolled in a writing course and a night class, History of the Vietnam War. For years I studied that debacle from a military point of view; now I looked forward to gaining insights on the political aspect of that mess.

The course turned out to be far and away the most in-depth and detailed (and truthful) examination of that part of our history I have ever seen or heard of. A fellow named Mike taught the class, assisted by Rob (we were all on a first-name basis here). Both were so good and their presentations so in harmony it was sometimes hard to tell which teacher was the official head honcho. Rob was an ex-Marine, a survivor of the Battle of Hue, that infamous carnage of the Tet Offensive of '68.

Mike brought in a phenomenal array of guest speakers: field grunts, pilots, special operations experts, ex-CIA agents, nurses. Most of the class were veterans, junior and senior high teachers, and a few students whose fathers were Nam vets who wouldn't talk to their kids about the war.

Rob asked me to "teach" a couple of three-hour class sessions. I gladly accepted; for, while most veterans refrain from public comment because the topic opens too many wounds, I felt it imperative for *someone* to step forward and do it. Besides, having spoken to so many high school classes with the VVA guys in New Jersey, I felt comfortable and competent as a guest teacher.

Never have I been involved in such an emotional class. Nothing was untouchable or unassailable, with one exception: Bad rapping of veterans for the war and the events of it was not allowed. We dwelt on controversies like the My-Lai massacre; but finger-pointing and blaming of ordinary foot soldiers was absolutely forbidden. Mike tolerated none of the sixties-type anti-veteran trash.

This was not the traditional name-date-place type of canned history course. He required students to research, to draw conclusions and support them. His teaching style required students to do something they weren't used to doing: they had to think and analyze. It led to heated discussions, to challenging one another and defending one's own positions. It also created the full gambit of emotion. Some burst out crying, others laughed uncontrollably. This was, without any doubt, one intense class.

Mike understood my pain and my whole physical problem caused by the Crohn's. Having colon cancer himself, Mike had similar problems. To him, teaching was a mission and he would teach until the end.

Frequently, Mike and I discussed my escapades with the VA. "I've seen many vets screwed by the system," he told me once. "Most of them just gave up. Don't you give up, Chuck." Mike was a model example of not giving up. I took inspiration from him.

In early May I called the Board of Veterans Appeals in D.C. to find out if the written transcript of my hearing was available yet. I gave the secretary my claim number and hearing date and I heard keys clicking as she searched for me in her computer.

"Not only is the written transcript available, but a decision has been made," she said. "Have you received your letter of notification?"

When I told her I had not, she asked, "Would you like to know what the decision was?"

"Well, naturally I'd like to know, if you can tell me."

I held my breath while I heard keys clicking again. I felt like a man accused of a crime he didn't commit waiting for the jury's verdict. I wanted to know but I was afraid to find out.

"Nine out of ten times I have to give bad news. ..." My stomach sank.

"... But this time it's good. ..."

My stomach rose.

"Your appeal to the BVA on March 28 was approved and granted in your favor."

All of me went nuts. This was too good to believe. I wanted to kiss the messenger. Right through the phone line. Clear across the continent.

The secretary said, "I don't know why you didn't receive your copy of the board's decision, but I'll send one if you would like. . . . Okay, I'll put it in today's mail. Let me confirm your current address. . . ."

I received my official copy the following Tuesday. I was enthralled with it. I won, I won, I won! The battle had been waged for just over eight years, but at last I was vindicated.

The best part of the letter was where the VA admitted they were "clearly and unmistakably in error." It felt *so good* to see them eating crow.

16 May 1989

Dear Mr. Lewis:

The Board has made its decision on the appeal in this case. I am enclosing a copy, which is self-explanatory. Your records are being returned to the office which has jurisdiction over your claim.

THE ISSUE

Entitlement to an effective date earlier than March 2, 1987, for the grant of service connection for a gastrointestinal disability, currently diagnosed as Crohn's disease.

CONCLUSIONS OF LAW

1. The rating action of July 1981, denying the veteran's claim for service connection for a gastrointestinal disability, was clearly and unmistakably in error; the grant of service connection for a gastrointestinal disability based on the veteran's application for service connection received by the VA in January 1981 is warranted.

2. An effective date of January 15, 1981 is warranted for the veteran's service-connected gastrointestinal disability, currently diagnosed as Crohn's disease.

ORDER

An effective date of January 15, 1981 for service connection for a gastrointestinal disability, currently diagnosed as Crohn's disease, is granted.

I hugged my mom. I called Mike and Rob. I told my friends. Then I sat back to wait for the regional office in New Jersey to calculate my award and send me my check. That would probably take a couple more weeks. But, oh well, hell, I'd waited over eight years, a couple more weeks won't matter.

I needed to have my files in the region of my residence — but I wasn't about to touch one hair on their head until after I got my award settlement. No use getting the regional offices screwed up and delaying me another year or two. After I got my award, *then* I would have my files transferred to Seattle and get on with the rest of my claim.

Six weeks later I still had heard nothing from the New Jersey Regional office. On June 20 I called New Jersey and asked about the status of my claim.

The guy I talked to said they couldn't find my records.

"Wait a minute. The Board of Appeals sent my records to your office on the nineteenth of May. Now they are somewhere in your system and I expect someone to find them and get back in touch with me."

On June 27 I called them back. The response was still the same: My records could not be found.

On Monday, July 3, I received a letter from New Jersey. It was dated June 29. That means that while my records were supposedly lost, they were actually in the office of the adjudicator. The lying bastards were either too lazy to search or they were just plain bullshitting me.

But this was not the letter the secretary told me I should be receiving.

> This refers to the Board of Veterans Appeals decision dated May 16, 1989.
>
> Although service connection has been granted for Crohn's disease effective January 15, 1981 with a 10 percent evaluation with a 30 percent evaluation from April 1, 1987, no change is warranted in the combined disability ratings for all your conditions. Your combined disability rating is still 40 percent from January 15, 1981, and 60 percent from April 1, 1987. You will continue to receive compensation benefits as before.

This was simply insane. The BVA awards me a 30 percent rating and the regional office decides to give me TEN percent? The regional office overturns a decision from the, quote, highest decision-making body available to veterans? And that, of course, saves the VA a chunk of money. What the hell is going on?

The BVA stated that my claim for retroactive benefits back to 1981 was justified. Newark had awarded me the thirty percent rating, and that rating had never been modified or rescinded. Since that is the only one ever given, the VA is required to use it as the basis for my retroactive pay and benefits. There had been no other physical exam, so there is absolutely no other base for the VA's rating. So how the hell can the VA Regional Office give me a rating of ten percent? All they have for evidence and decision making is the standard disability complaint I have provided all these years.

I wanted answers and I wanted them right now. I got on the phone, knowing I was about to put my mom's phone bill right through the roof.

I called the VA Regional Office in Newark and demanded to speak to the top honcho in that august institution. He told me the ten percent rating was "ordered by the Board of Veterans Appeals."

"I have trouble believing that. If the BVA made such a decision it would have said so in my Statement of Findings and Decision."

"Well, Mr. Lewis, not all information is necessarily included in documents we send out."

"Right. I'm only the claimant. Veterans aren't entitled to know what's in their files, what's in those mysterious documents you don't want us to see, or what's in those decisions you make about their lives. Frankly, sir, all this is bullshit. But I am not ready to roll over and die; you can be sure I will be in touch with you again soon."

My next call was to the BVA in Washington, and again I demanded to talk to a supervisor. He claimed to be as baffled about the ten percent rating as I was. But not baffled enough to go searching for some how-comes and whys. "All the information pertaining to your claim is included in your Statement of Decision," he said. "There is no need for me to question the New Jersey regional office."

Now it's time to call Newark again. I get to talk to yet another person, go through the whole four-reel show again.

And Mr. Yet Another Person says the same thing: "The BVA made the decision."

"Don't give me that shit. I just got off the phone with the BVA in Washington and they had no idea where you guys in Newark came up with the ten percent rating."

Silence. I feared I had been cut off. The next thing I knew I was talking to still one more Yet Another Person. It was obvious the worms were crawling out of this opened can and nobody wanted to touch them.

For the fourth time I told the story.

The fourth guy on the phone tut-tutted in phony sympathy but said there was little he could do

"Yes, there is. Let's talk about the ten percent issue. The Board of Appeals said the effective date of the award was to be January 1981."

"Well, we issued the new rating based on your 1981 physical exam. So I guess that does make 1981 the effective date."

"This has obviously gotten muddled in some people's minds. I'm clear on it, and so is the Board of Appeals. So I guess you're the one that needs help. I'm going to spell it out, and you try to follow." I doubted anyone in Newark had the intellect to get it, but I was going to give it to him anyway.

"Letter A. The VA did not evaluate me for Crohn's disease in 1981. You can't just make up things and say they happened.

"Letter B. I was denied entitlements from the start because of the VA's failure to put it in writing that I had Crohn's.

"Letter C. The Veterans Board of Appeals adjudicated that the VA's failure to note the presence of Crohn's disease in 1981 was, quote, *clearly and mistakenly in error.*

"Letter D. The paper titled Issue of the Claim specifically orders the current rating decision to be made retroactive to 1981.

"Letter E. The thirty percent retroactive rating is very explicit.

"Letter F. The Board of Veterans Appeals is supposed to be the highest adjudicating body of the Veterans Administration. The Newark Veterans Administration Regional Office overturning a Appeals Board decision is about as moral as a Night Court judge flipping off the Chief Justice. But then, according to the VA, the system *really works.*"

The VA regional office in Newark had a very short and simple response: "If you don't like this decision, file another appeal."

Next I called the Board of Veterans Appeals — again — and questioned about the ethics and legality of the VARO ignoring the Board's decision and inventing their own. I was told that the BVA had no real legal jurisdiction over the regional offices' decisions.

"Then what is your purpose for being?" I asked. "A decision making body whose decisions can be ignored? That seems to translate to a building full of government-salaried bureaucrats with no authority and no job descriptions."

"I don't have any answers to those questions," admitted the fellow. "But if you request another hearing, we can hope to eliminate some of the loopholes the regional offices use.

I spoke with someone else somewhere else — I was being transferred about every two sentences and it was impossible to keep track of where I was or to whom I spoke. The bottom line was: I needed to file another appeal — although along the way someone who told me he'd "do what he could" for me but his "authority is such matters is extremely limited." By now I understood the plain-English translation of that: Nobody does anything and the vet goes away.

The only reason I got off the phone was that it was five o'clock on the East Coast. By now the phone bill was going through the roof and so was I. All this was just inconceivable to me. I knew I still had to pursue the upgrade, but I really thought I had received an official letter saying this point, at least, was officially behind me. Now I am back at square one, point zero. Frustration just overwhelmed me.

Okay, all you Yet Another Do Nothing, Know Nothing Persons, the gauntlet is on the ground. I am still alive and breathing and as long as I am, I will continue to be in your faces. I will come up with the money to get back to D.C. for another hearing if I have to knock off a bank or a store.

The Fourth of July, 1989 was a day without meaning to me. I spent it inside a numb cloud of so-what.

On July fifth I called Ed Stevens. I figured my BVA rep ought to be able to suggest what I should do next. Hell, he's my representative — maybe he could even get this hassle with the regional office resolved.

Wrong again. Stevens wasn't working any harder these days than when he flubbed my case in the first place. "Nothing I can do," he said.

"You got what you appealed for, which was getting service connection for the Crohn's disease made retroactive to January of eighty-one," he said. "The thirty percent award was never part of the issue."

"Excuse me. Yes, it was. Plus a number of other items were issues, too — until you decided you could only handle one concept at a time. Between the moment of the hearing and the moment of now, you, Mr. Stevens, have changed your entire line. You begged me to stay for the hearing to get the retroactive award *and* the thirty percent rating because you said that getting *this* award would give me the finances to pursue the rest of my claim; you remember that? Or were you just passing the platitudes so I wouldn't kill you in the rage you put me in?"

Right now I wanted to kill him even deader than I should have killed him back then.

I spent the next couple of days doing the only thing I thought would do any good. I sat at the computer my parents bought me and started hammering out letters to all the congressmen and senators who had been involved in my case, plus the Washington state delegation.

In March, 1989 the Congress created the Department of Veterans Affairs and its secretary became part of the President's Cabinet. Some of the traditional veterans' organizations had sided with the VA in opposing this move: it opened the VA to more scrutiny. Not much; but at least a little accountability was now written in. At any rate, I wrote a heated letter to Edward J. Derwinski, President Bush's appointee as first secretary of the new cabinet-level department.

The quickest way to get the most action is to threaten an individual's power. Frankly, the new Secretary was the head of an agency that had no power and in which all divisions were equally impotent. "The biggest question," I wrote, "is why can the VAROs read anything they wish into a Board of Appeals decision, and the veteran's only recourse is to file another appeal? This is a waste of taxpayer money and board members' time. It also denies the veteran a timely resolution to his claim and prolongs his situation. At this stage of things the veteran is normally in a severe situation, anyway, without his public servants adding to it."

While I was about it I sent the same letter to President Bush. And with all my letters, I included copies of my past correspondence with legislators and documents from the VA.

Naturally I needed a friend with a big ear. I called Stumpy. He told me he had just completed his training course and was now a service representative for Vietnam Veterans of America. I related the latest episode, complete with the good four-letter words and angry sound bites. Stumpy, bless his heart for being no-baloney frank and forthright, said, "You just been fucked again by the system."

Stumpy reminded me of the Judicial Review legislation recently enacted. "You may be one of the first cases heard by the new Judicial Review Board," he said. "Your case is definitely valid."

Stumpy is a brilliant and good man who not only understands the veteran but he understands the system. But until the VA and all its in-cahoots brethren do some serious housecleaning, no individual will be able to change it, no matter his intellect and empathy. So I said, "The new court only allows me to argue points of law and to ascertain if my rights have been violated. My case would still be remanded back to the VA for reconsideration. At which time they could do it all again in a different way, just like Newark changed their own rules in the middle of their act. This could end up being an endless cycle."

Stumpy agreed. "That's why we must continue to lobby for the CVA to have more power and authority."

He approved my letter-writing campaign. He said he would represent me if I went back to Washington for another Board of Veterans Appeals hearing. I told him I wouldn't want anyone else.

"These bureaucratic agencies claim they're saving taxpayers money," I told Stumpy. "Considering staff salaries and perks, paper, phone calls, and having to build buildings for people to do nothing in, I figure that in the eight-plus years this has been dragging out, the VA must have spent about sixty thousand bucks to keep me from getting less than three hundred a month."

In August the Chief of Staff of the Secretary of the Department of Veterans Affairs responded to my letters to President Bush and Secretary Derwinski. It was couched in the strange language of Bureauboggle Formalese, but in plain English it meant *Your case is just tough stuff. If you don't like the way we do things then refile your claim.* This discourteous, uncaring bit of terse verse was the best-writing effort of the highest office in the cabinet-level Department of Veterans Affairs.

On August 30 the Seattle Regional Office finally received my records from Newark — more than a month after Newark got the transfer order. Seattle said they would review my file and "get in touch" me.

The approach of Labor Day meant summer's end. Obviously I wasn't to see Andrea this year. Somehow I had this silly notion that Tina would honor her promise to let Andrea spend some of her summer with me; but true to herself, Tina refused to allow her to come. Tina said she would let Andrea come to Seattle for Christmas. I didn't believe her for a minute, but nevertheless I stashed every piece of loose change in a jar I labeled Andrea's Trip.

39

On the first of September the local newspaper came to my mom's apartment for a story on me and my housing situation. I carefully explained how the VA was the cause of my homelessness, and I seized the opportunity to mention that nearly thirty percent of the nation's homeless are veterans. Only a smidge of my story was included in the printed article, but it was enough for the Housing Authority to get me an apartment. My rent, $157 a month, was based on my current income from the VA. That was not a net setback for me, because I had been paying my parents about the same sum.

Fall quarter began at GRCC. Mike's cancer progressed. The college administration generously allowed him to continue teaching, but Mike had to curtail his schedule: Two weeks on, two off. Stan was employed to teach during Mike's off weeks, and Rob continued assisting on a volunteer basis. As teacher, assistant, and man Friday, Stan, Rob, and I had a great time. We were strongly wavelengthed together and shared a common mission.

Having served in Vietnam, Stan had seen the VA's mistreatment of veterans, and he made that the subject of the final two class sessions. Students were amazed and shocked by the system's atrocities. We did nothing to soothe them.

I told the group why, according to the government, Agent Orange "had no known detrimental effects on humans." I told the students, "The truth is, this country is governed by Political Action Committees. Each PAC has its own axes, its own agendas, and PACs buy the politicians. If you kids have idealistic notions that you can't buy votes, let me tell you that a quarter million dollars donated to a candidate's campaign fund makes the candidate eternally committed to the cause of the donor.

"Chemical companies who paid to get Senator Blowhard elected, for example, now own Senator Blowhard. Ergo, Agent Orange's side effects — no such thing, announce the chemists' elected mouthpieces.

"Some changes have been made," I told the collegians. "Giving the DVA Cabinet status. Establishing the Court of Veterans Appeals. Training Vietnam vets to represent their peers (I told the class about Stumpy). But changes occur far too late. I want a new Wall in Washington, D.C. dedicated to veterans whose death was from Agent Orange, or suicide, or from the VA's neglect. We can call it The Wall of Shame."

In November I was notified that my GI Bill education benefits would be slashed on January 1, 1990. This would be my last quarter at the current rate — the rate the government promised to maintain for ten years past discharge. By the ten-year formula, I was entitled to schooling until January, 1991. Of course I could stay in school, but with lower payments. This is another Congressional attempt to save money at the expense of veterans.

The GI Bill was changed as a result of legislation coming out of the House Committee on Veterans Affairs, ostensibly hawked in the name of saving taxpayer dollars. The truth of it is it was a plain-old ego trip for the House Committee chairman. A lawmaker writes up a bill and he gets his name on it. The Montgomery GI Bill, the Montgomery Judicial Review Act. Would he be endowed with the Montgomery Veterans Administration, too?

In November I accepted the inevitable and filed for a new hearing. Christ, this wasn't ever going to end. Before I formally filed my appeal, I contacted Stumpy to see if the VA recognized any service reps in the Seattle area. The final choice was a fellow named George Simpson from the American Legion. I would use a local rep for the preliminary stage of the process, but if I went back to D.C. for a Judicial Review Board hearing, it would be side by side and back to back with Stumpy.

Beth, a student in my class, skipped school to drive me to Seattle to meet with George Simpson. With a nursing degree and a year of hospital experience behind her, Beth was now studying to be an occupational therapist. She also cared for a family member with Crohn's disease, so we were kindreds.

George went over my file with me, making sure he had all the information and that he understood every speck of it. He was amazed by the whole history and handling — no, mishandling — of my claim, and was as confused as I about how Newark came the rating decision they made.

As we left the Federal Building I spotted the Federal Book Store on the first floor. I went in to peruse. And found a lost gold mine. There on the shelf in front of me was a stack of volumes called *Code of Federal Regulations (CFR)*. Among them was CFR Title 38 Parts 0 to 17 and 18 to End. This is the VA's bible. I had fifty dollars to last me another two weeks, and I needed to pay for our parking. But I gladly paid the forty dollars for those two books. In my own hot little hands, I had the rules and regulations the VA does not want veterans to see. I now had the VA by the gonads.

I had the first book open before we were out of the parking lot. As we rolled south on I-5, I gleefully went nuts finding arguable points of contention with almost everything the VA had done in the past. Beth smiled and nodded as I excitedly quoted stuff which I knew would make the difference between winning my next appeal or losing it. These books were a coup! I was about to have fun with the VA now. The specifics went over Beth's head because she didn't understand the details of my babbling, but my glee and excitement kind of flowed over to her.

As I analyzed the books, I figured out: (A) They were typical government work, written for anyone with a moron factor of four to understand. (B) For every rule there is a counter rule . . . so (C) Make your interpretation of the rules seem stronger than the counter rule. He who argues loudest and quotes the most rules wins.

"Why did you wait so long to buy these books?" Beth asked, laughing.

"Well, first off, nobody puts them in out in plain sight to be bought. And the VA and its representatives sure don't want to recommend them."

I hung a Post-It Note on my brain to remind myself to tell everyone in my class about the Code of Federal Regulations books. And tell Stumpy, so he can pass the word to the guys in the chapter. Stumpy could tell them the CFRs are in federal book stores, or in reference sections of larger libraries.

After Beth dropped me off at home I brewed up some fresh coffee and hit the books, studying like I was preparing for a bar exam. First I focused on disability compensation and the various levels of awards. For a medical problem with this symptom it's a twenty percent rating; for the same problem with *these* symptoms it might be a forty percent.

Thanks to these books, never again would I discuss my claim in layman's terms. Now I will use the VA's language and quote its own regulations to its agents. My new knowledge also meant I will require George Simpson to discuss my case on a professional level. No longer will I accept anyone's talking down to me, trying to editorialize regulations that I'm not allowed to read for myself.

Beth and I were getting pretty close . . . but, see . . . well, the thing is: Beth wasn't the only one! Ruth is a smart, compassionate, living doll whom I also met at college. I liked, admired, respected, and adored both of them, and it wasn't all chemistry-and-hormones: with each there was a base of solid friendship. I took each of them out and had a hell of a good time. Here I was just out of a relationship that emotionally busted me; now I am having a great time with *two* women. If I weren't fearful of involvement, I could have been very happy with either of these terrific women; but I was scared of commitment and a long time away from being ready for anything permanent.

The last holiday season of the new decade passed in a blur of joy, despair, and confusion.

I was single and my own person.

Through my college class, I was contributing to society.

Tina did not allow Andrea to come for Christmas, just as Voice On My Shoulder kept trying me to prepare for. I knew that any Christmas presents I sent Andrea would be intercepted by her grandparents and discarded; so I took the money in Andrea's Trip jar and bought her a savings bond. I did not send it to her; I kept it with my important papers.

I had no money. But on the bright side of that, Tina wasn't around to blow what I didn't have.

I devoted time to Beth and Ruth both. Boy, this stuff of having two beautiful women is hard to work out!

Finally, the holidays were over and we stepped into a new decade.

40

On January 8, 1990 I received a letter from the VA.

> You have filed a Notice of Disagreement with our action on your claim, the first step in appealing to the Board of Veterans Appeals. This letter and attachments give you very important information. Please read them carefully.
>
> If we do not hear from you in 60 days, we will assume you do not intend to complete your appeal and we will close our record. If you are required more time, please let us know within 60 days.

So the VA was still up to its "if we do not hear from you" ploy. Still hoping letters get lost and they can get out of as much work as they can.

Other than that, this letter made me happy. First, it came much sooner than I expected. And it included a lot more information than the VA generally provided. Maybe my hell- raising at those hearings had the VA operating in a little better manner.

The other thing that made me happy was, thanks to the Code of Federal Regulations, I knew the VA conveniently left out some details, and I knew what they were and where to find them to quote them back. According to 38 CFR 1.102:

> When reasonable doubt arises regarding service origin, the degree of disability, or any other point, such doubt will be resolved in favor of the claimant. A reasonable doubt means a substantial doubt and one within the range of probability as distinguished from speculation or remote possibility.
>
> . . . Mere suspicion or doubt as to the truth of any statements submitted ... is not justifiable basis for

> denying the application ... The reasonable doubt doctrine is also applicable even in the absence of official records, particularly if the basic incident allegedly arose under combat or similar strenuous conditions, and is consistent with the probable results of such known hardships.

Two days later I received another letter from the VA. It told me to show up at the regional office in Seattle at 0900 hours on March 12, 1990 for "the hearing you requested."

I called George Simpson. "Help me understand what's going on here," I said. "I get a letter on January eighth telling me I'll appear before the Board of Veterans Appeals in D.C. On January tenth I get a letter telling me my hearing will be held here. What's the deal?"

"The Seattle office felt we could handle your appeal locally. And your hearing date will be much sooner here."

"I can go along with that if the hearing addresses every single issue I put on the table. All present issues and all past ones. No ambiguous rulings."

"We can do that."

Okay, March 12, 1990 it will be. My day for another chance at justice. I hit the Code of Federal Regs books again for more research.

My Crohn's condition was going downhill fast and I wasn't keeping up in school. Mike, who knew everyone worth knowing, did his best to help me get a job, but nothing ever panned out.

Beth and Ruth both noticed my deteriorating physical condition and both tried to get me to go to the hospital. I wouldn't. I wouldn't go to the VA. I have no insurance for a civilian doctor, and I damn sure can't pay the bill in cash.

Mike continued to worsen and he spent more and more time at home. Instead of working with Mike, the school's administration did everything it could to drive him away. The school's president was a man with a master's in business administration who knew nothing of education or the learning process.

Mike, on the other hand, was the consummate educator, thoroughly committed to his students and his academic discipline. To Mike, history was constant. What happened, happened. Who was there, was there. You couldn't go back and put people there who were not, nor delete those who were. I admired Mike's integrity as an educator and his commitment to his family. And for his courage in fighting for two things at once. His life. Quality education.

To his credit, Mike allowed dissentious discussions, and so did Stan, Rob, and I. Pam was one of the dissenters, a serious anti-war activist. Her point of view was extremely important to the total context of the Vietnam war, for the history of the Vietnam War cannot be addressed without including the anti-war movement.

Rob and I were openly hostile to her, however, because we understood her to be blaming the foot soldier personally for everything that went wrong with the war. Pam, on the other hand, thought we were attacking her personally for the anti-war movement. But then, we had our own experiences on our side. Veterans felt that the movement was specifically aimed at us instead of the decision makers.

Pam raised hell with the military, personally and as an entity, for participating in the destruction of life, property, and the environment. She was correct that those things happened; they are undeniable facts of war. She believed in alternative methods of settling conflicts. But dammit, that is the responsibility of a country's leaders. The soldier in Vietnam was in a particularly rock-hard place situation: If he acted on his moral and political beliefs, he got court martialed. If he followed orders, he got ostracized and spat upon when he returned home. A key point that civilians in the "peace" movement forget is: the military does not act on its own. It takes its orders from the Commander in Chief (the President) and the Congress.

From those stormy sessions, something happened which I never thought could: I became friends with an anti-Vietnam war activist. After Pam, Rob, and I each set all our plates on the table, we better understood the other's stand. No one changed anyone's mind: we agreed to disagree. After that we each discovered that the other side's money bought just as good a beer as ours.

An All-American Horsepower team declared their intent to go to the March 12 hearing in Seattle to testify on my behalf. Beth, Ruth, Stan, Rob, and Janet.

Janet I had known since 1982, when we started college together. She had been known to stick up for me publicly when

Tina was doing some of her rumor-mongering; and I, along with Rob and a couple of others, had found out who slashed Janet's tires and we had gleefully taken revenge by spray painting the spendy little sports car his daddy got him for graduation, supergluing the locks, and pin-holing the valve stems of the tires. With Janet and Rob and me, nobody messed with one of us without having to deal with all three.

While I was in New Jersey, Janet was the faultless one in a traffic accident that broke her neck and left her right arm paralyzed. True to our past history, she made it clear she would be there for the hearing and "we'll kick some VA ass, man."

Having Mike testify for me would be like bringing a pair of aces up each sleeve. Mike, the most intellectual individual I have ever had the privilege of calling my friend, would address the VA with language and thought processes that would whiz right over the heads of the board members. He exuded presence and authority when he got his crank turned. But he steadily grew worse and there was simply no way I would ask him to expend the last of his strength on me. His family needed that strength more.

Rob and I went to visit Mike one afternoon in February, and we left brooding, knowing he would not make it through the summer.

The guys in the VVA chapter back in New Jersey undertook a writing campaign and furnished me with an armload of letters for the hearing board's record. Ted, still a loyal friend, added his. My ammunition was mounting.

Another little known regulation which the VA conveniently keeps to itself states that veterans are allowed to present written statements by third party witnesses to support their claim. According to CFR 38, 3.200, both oral and written testimony "presented by the claimant or in his behalf for the purpose of establishing a claim for service connection" are acceptable, provided such testimony is "certified or under oath or affirmation. Well, hell, Stumpy's a notary public. My VVA brothers hand Stumpy a letter, he pa-choonks it with his notary's seal, and it's legally sworn.

Stumpy and I agreed to keep the tide contained at under fifty this time, but if I need to go yet another round, I figure to overwhelm the VA with hundreds of letters from supporters.

As I prepared myself, I needed to discuss a couple of questions with George. When I called his office I was told he had been transferred to eastern Washington.

Oh, SHIT. Here we go again.

Visions of getting screwed up by another service rep warp-speeded past me. Here I am at the eleventh hour and I find my service rep is gone without so much as a "Kiss me, sucker," or "Good luck, I turned your case over to Someone."

I was call-forwarded to a man named I Am Alan And I'll Be Your New Service Representative. He assured me he could put everything together by March 12.

So if he's so sincere why didn't he make any effort to contact you the minute George bailed out? Why didn't George contact you himself?

"Let's discuss your case, see what we have and what I can do," Alan said.

"Tell you what, Alan. Let's hang up and you call me back in five seconds. We'll talk on your dime."

We did and he did and we spent an hour discussing my case on his dime. He seemed genuine — but then, so did Ed and George and all the others at first. Accordingly, I set my deck face-up on the table.

"I want to make this real clear," I told Alan. "I don't need any more shit pulled on me like Ed and the DAV pulled at the Board of Appeals hearing. I want this to be the end of it all." In fact I wanted this to end it all so much that I would be willing to make a compromise on the entitlement if it would get this insane frustration over with. But that was not something I was about to say aloud to anyone.

Alan set up a meeting for the following week.

I continued poring over the Code of Federal Regulations manuals, looking for things to shore up my case, however small or borderline iffy they may be. I found one that I doubted really applied to me, but decided to go for it anyway.

According to CFR 38 3.801, a veteran is entitled to an additional allowance for clothing when ". . . the veteran wears or uses certain prosthetic or orthopedic appliances which tend to wear or tear clothing (including a wheelchair) ... "

I have no orthopedic or prosthetic devices. However, I do tend to ruin a lot of clothing because of the uncontrolled chronic diarrhea. I figured that the VA, being so tied to the literal, would deny me on the issue. Nevertheless, I incorporated it into my request, hoping to draw the Board's attention to other ways a disability can ruin clothing. This also enabled me to demonstrate a dramatic effect of my diarrhea problem.

I also prepared my written statement for the record that included sixteen different posts and paragraphs from the regulations that directly applied to my case — in addition to the regulations that spell out my rights of appeal. No wonder the VA doesn't want vets to get their hands on those books.

My written statement of case included a list of problems I have in living with the Crohn's disease — eleven of them, plus the notation: "Depends undergarments do not absorb diarrhea."

After the simple A, B, C listing, I explained my medical problems in greater detail.

I described the havoc that all this has created in my personal life and employment opportunities.

I attacked the New Jersey Regional Office's overturning the Board of Appeals and demoting me to a ten percent rating.

Altogether I had a sixteen-page statement which I felt more than amply presented my case.

I figured that with my statement, plus my records, which were updated and current (provided no papers got deleted from my file), plus oral testimony and all the letters from my battalion of friends, I had an open and shut case.

Except nothing is open and shut with the VA. Racking my meager mental abilities, I searched for the one loophole the VA might find to use against me. I trusted that fine upstanding organization about as far as I could throw the building it occupied.

Finally, I couldn't think of one other scrap of information to include. I felt pretty good about what I had put together.

Rob got his PTSD physical scheduled at long last ... for March 12. Dear friend that he was, he offered to have his ordeal rescheduled so he could testify at my hearing as we planned. I told him no way. I of all people knew how difficult it was to get through the VA's doorway, and I would absolutely not jeopardize his chances to get his own claim resolved. Cross off Rob's testimony.

41

Beth came to my rescue again and drove me into Seattle to meet with Alan at the American Legion Service Rep Office. I scoped out good karma with him, just as I had with George.

Getting right to the point, I showed Alan the written statement I prepared. The farther he read, the more stunned he looked.

"All the regulations you've quoted . . . How did you get that information?"

"Just walked into the bookstore downstairs and bought the Code of Federal Regulations," I said matter-of-factly.

A half scared, half surprised expression crossed his face, which he quickly rearranged into a lame smile.

"I got fed up with the VA's habit of not telling me the rules, and of misapplying them to suit their own incompetence and indifference," I explained. "I got the books so I could build my own case."

"But you don't need to go to all that work. That's why there are service reps," Alan said, taken aback.

I laid into him over that. "Service reps are adept at keeping veterans in the dark. The ones I've dealt with over the past nine years neglected to inform me about regulations I found by myself. Why is that the Code is kept so secret? Why does the VA go to such extremes to keep veterans from reading the book? Hell, in nine years nobody even *told* me there was such a thing."

Alan made a few feeble attempts at covering the VA's ass. I wasn't up for any more of that nonsense, and I told him so.

Then I said, "Now that you clearly understand that I know what the VA has been doing all these years, let us proceed with this case like two professional people working together. If I have overlooked any point at all, or if I have any fact not entirely accurate, or if there is a single T not crossed or an I not dotted, you will inform me and it will be corrected. I am going to win this case this time, and as my service representative, you will be responsible for the outcome."

By the conclusion of our meeting I was reasonably satisfied that Alan would do what no one else who represented me had done: He would help me win and bring this battle to an end.

The following weekend I had my worst-ever flare-up of Crohn's disease. The cramps were awesome. I spent as much time on the pot as off.

At ten o'clock, as I walked down the stairs to watch the news, an excruciating cramp seized me. As I began teetering I jumped to the bottom of the stairs to avoid taking a fall. Instead of landing on my feet, I alighted on the side of my ankle. I heard the *pop* and I felt the bone snap as I bounced off the door at the bottom of the stairs.

I dragged myself to the phone to try to find someone to take me to the hospital. I spent three hours on the phone, foot elevated and iced, without raising anyone. Well ... Friday night ... out doing the town.

I spent the night in serious pain, dragging myself between toilet and bed. First, though, came the agony of getting back up the stairs to get to the bedroom.

At 1:30 Saturday afternoon, I finally reached Beth. She hurried to the apartment, gave me what-for for not waking her in the night, helped me drag myself to her car, and sped to the VA hospital.

I went straight to the emergency room. The main-desk clerk punched my information into the computer. Then she turned to me with disdain on her face.

"You are not a veteran," she fairly sneered.

Later I discovered that the computer at the VA hospital doesn't talk to the ones in VA offices. How easily remedied, and how inexcusably, negligently inefficient!

Finally I was admitted because I carried a wallet size copy of my discharge papers. But first the clerk required me to fill out several forms. All this time I was left standing on the foot that was not hanging loose on my leg. I was not offered a wheel chair, nor was I allowed to be seated to fill out the forms.

X-rays showed that not only was the ankle broken, but there was almost a half inch separation of the bone. The doctor could only apply a splint because the swelling was so prominent. When the swelling subsided I would have to go back for a proper cast. Then he sent me home with a bottle of pain pills. That inefficient institution didn't even have crutches. I had to wait for those until Monday, when I got the cast put on.

I didn't go back for the crutches. My mom had a pair I used instead.

It was an agonizing extreme to go to find a silver lining, but I would use the incident to add credence to my case. I adamantly insisted the doctor note in my medical records that my fall was caused by severe pain and cramping during an episode of Crohn's disease. That was a point I had learned the hard way, to document anything that happened as a result of a side effect of the primary condition.

On Thursday evening two weeks later, a member of the VA Adjudication Department called with some questions. What a startle! Never once in nine years had I spoken to anyone in the adjudication department. These guys are essentially unreachable. Why this contact now? Two hours past quitting time, yet. *What shoe is he going to drop on you, Lewis?*

With all courtesy, he asked for some clarifications. I certainly was willing to talk with him. That was it. No surprises.

My hearing was Tuesday. On Friday evening, I was horrified to realized I still had not gotten the letter from the VV. chapter in Jersey. In a panic, I called Jay to find out what happened to all that support I was promised.

As it turned out, Jack, who was appointed guardian of the letter, had forgotten to mail it.

Even if Jack mailed it that very second, there wasn't a prayer of a chance I'd get it in time for the hearing. "I'll fax it," Jack said.

Very quickly I located a public fax machine at a nearby pharmacy, then called Jack with its phone number. For an hour or so there was a lot of scurrying around in Jersey and in Cent, Washington ... but I got the fax. It was just spewing out of the machine when I raced into the pharmacy — five minutes before it closed for the weekend.

The letter wasn't as strong as I hoped, but it carried several points that would help me. Most significant was the narrative from chapter members who worked for the New Jersey Department of Labor who attempted to help me find a job. Their expert opinion was that as a direct result of Crohn's disease, I am unemployable.

They attributed the disintegration of my marriage to the unemployability.

They noted I could not fully participate in chapter events because of chronic diarrhea which is a symptom of Crohn's.

Ruth's bold, from-the-hip statement attacked the issue head on.

TO WHOM IT MAY CONCERN:

I am writing this letter to the appropriate officials in the Department of Veterans Affairs, on behalf of Charles A. Lewis.

While Mr. Lewis was assisting me with some shopping on 6 Jan. 1990 at a local department store, he had a spontaneous attack of his Crohn's disease, and had a bowel movement in his pants while in the store. Mr. Lawrence could not make it to the restroom, it happened so fast.

It goes without saying this was excruciatingly embarrassing for him, as it was for myself who was accompanying. It was far from a comfortable drive home to say the least.

I am writing this to testify that he does indeed have this problem, and to support him in his case and claim for his disability. Mr. Lewis incurred this problem while he was still in the service. His condition is so severe that he can not get a job because of it. It is not his fault he has a medical condition that inhibits him socially, nor is it his fault that employers feel they can not deal with the condition.

I do know his self esteem has suffered drastically because of the way he has had to lead his life for almost a full decade. It is no surprise that on several occasions he has suggested suicide. It is a shame that a veteran like Mr. Lewis must suffer and do without the basic security of life simply because his problem does not totally meet the criteria established in your regulations.

Thank you.

Ruth's letter spoke of my present problem. The one from Ted took my Crohn's history clear back to 1981. Together, the two statements ought to give the board a picture of both the duration and progress of my condition, and of its severity.

So. Now all my papers, documents, and records were ready. A squadron of people ready to show up, speak up, and support me. All right, Department of Veterans Affairs ... bring in your clowns.

The heavy-hitting team of horsepower who promised to show up at my hearing ... didn't.

Stan couldn't get off work.

Ruth got sick.

Janet just flat copped out. That was a devastating blow, though more personally than hearing-wise. I had known her for over ten years. But now, she of shared pranks and of philosophies in common, now she went around telling our friends — whom we shared in common as well — she really didn't know me well enough to testify on my behalf.

But Beth was there, she, and the strong, by-the-rulebook case I had prepared, and my artillery of written statements bearing so many signatures. My doctor in Jersey furnished the statement from the Agent Orange Commission. The chief of the gastrointestinal division of the VA hospital in Seattle prepared a statement describing Crohn's disease and its related problems, and explaining the difference between Crohn's and ulcerative colitis. "Colitis, possibly" was my original diagnosis; and in all these years, the VA had never gotten it through its collective head that: One, it was a misdiagnosis in the first place, and Two, the two are different.

The veteran must provide an awesome amount of evidence to support his claim — despite the misnamed "friendly, casual atmosphere" of the hearings. The VA promotes its hearings as "non-adversarial," and that misleads the poor slob who hasn't been through the process. Veterans must go to the extreme to support their claims. All right, Mr. Hearing Board and Associates, I am prepared in the extreme.

It was now time to confront the dragon.

Beth and I arrived at Alan's office right on schedule. Alan laid out the final plan of attack. He said he was so impressed with my written statement that after his opening and general introductions, he would turn the presentation over to me. I would present the majority of my case myself, because, as he said, who knew better than I what to say and what to ask?

I got on my crutches and Alan, Beth, and I went upstairs to meet the enemy.

The hearing was presided over by a sole and single adjudicator who introduced himself as Dave. He explained the procedure, concluding: "In the event you object to the decision of this hearing, Mr. Lewis, you will then be entitled to pursue your claim with the Board of Appeals. Further appeal would go to the Court of Veterans Appeals."

My insides smiled at the mention of the Court. Little did Dave know that, back in 1985, I was one of the original movers and supporters for forming the court. Little did he know, either, that if I had to take my case that far, my friend Stumpy would be there.

After our swearing-in, Alan overviewed the history of my case and told the adjudicator, one, two, three, A, B, C, what my claim asked for.

Then the floor was mine.

I chronicled my entire conflict with the VA to date. I detailed every wrong decision I contested. I documented every protest, citing by chapter and section the regulations in the Federal Code.

I challenged the previous Board of Veterans Appeals decision and explained how the regional office in New Jersey mishandled and botched it. Again, I cited specific small-print parentheses inside of footnotes to mini-micro-subsections to subchapters of the Federal Regs.

I enumerated how the disease closed me out of employment, and how the VA provided no kind of job search assistance, not even leads.

So that I wouldn't sound too combative, I excused the previous adjudicators' ignorance of my medical problem: My early records did not use the word *Crohn's*. Nor did the VA's guidebook explain the difference between Crohn's and ulcerative colitis. So I explained it.

I could not resist adding that in nine years, the VA had done little or nothing to help me. I said it unemotionally, a reporter reciting fact — for me, a triumph of restraint.

Beth's turn. When out of my house, did I hover around the restroom? Any knowledge of my having accidents in public? Could she attest to ways the disease affected my social, academic, and business dealings?

Dave, the adjudicator, asked a few questions about my social life and work history, and about Crohn's disease itself. Everything he asked had already been aired, and it was my impression that Dave was trying to educate himself about the condition to establish a proper decision in this case. And in others down the road.

After adjourning the hearing, Dave said, "Let's talk about your disability rating. Off the record." He turned off the recorder, dismissed the clerk, closed up all his folders and notebooks, pocketed his pen, and got out of the adjudicator's chair. His body language said "off the record."

"Combing all factors under consideration," I said, "my case honestly and legitimately deserves a one hundred percent rating on its own merit. If I have to, I will accept the hundred percent based on unemployability. Viewed that way, I really have a case for two times one hundred percent."

Dave left and returned with the form for requesting 100 percent disability based on unemployability. "Fill it out and return it," he said. "And, Mr. Lewis. Thank you for your fine presentation."

I was told that the tape had to be sent to Minneapolis for transcription, then sent to the adjudication department for a decision. About ninety days.

That's a screwed-up system. Send a tape halfway across the continent? Like nobody in all the Pacific Northwest knows how to listen and type the words. Yeah, but I feel pretty good about this one.

On the way home we stopped at a greaseburger pit so Beth could stoke up. She was raging-mad at Janet for copping out at the last minute. "After all her big talk the past few months. Going to write a letter, going to speak up in your defense. Going to save your case! Bull!" she snorted.

I was hurt by Janet's chickening out; I was truly emotionally wounded. Beth was plain-old livid. I tried placating her. "I think we made it without her," I told Beth.

42

Despite the confidence I conveyed to all my friends and classmates who asked about the hearing, it was easy to have inner jitters about anything involving the VA. Waiting for such an important decision about one's life can drive one nuts. I wanted the results yesterday ... but I feared knowing. Would I get another denial because of some bullshit loophole the VA makes up as it goes along? Or would I win and finally put all this to rest?

I called Stumpy and I called Tim, principally to let them know the hearing happened, that I thought their efforts on my behalf were fruitful, and that I appreciated their friendship and support. Both cautioned me not to expect too much until the award was in my hands. I already knew that.

Throughout the rest of the term I went to school as I was able and helped with the Vietnam history class as I could. By now Mike had grown so ill and weak he had all but relinquished his teaching duties. We had a special bond, Mike and I, and when he asked, I tried to make as if I had won my case because I didn't want him worrying about me.

Now hovering on death, he had more important things on his mind. Things like his wife and kids, who, always and until the end, came first. Things like his students and their pursuit of the truth of history. Mike had put his heart and soul into this class. He saw the Vietnam period tear this country apart, and he saw the need to have his program in place while the real questions needed answering. The amount of healing that took place in that classroom would be the envy of any vet's center rap group or counseling program. And I feared that after Mike was gone, the program would become just another boring, mundane history course.

The college administration was already looking for someone to take over Mike's class. Rob and Stan and I began lobbying for Stan to be named the official instructor. He had knowledge of the Vietnam war, both from the military and political sides. Besides that, he had the sheepskin that qualified him for the instructorship.

Except for grieving for Mike, I went through the following months on a high. With the companionship of some good friends, I enjoyed life, perhaps more than at any other time. *Friends.* So many good and loyal ones, on two coasts. The irony of it struck me, that the only person who didn't like and support me was: my wife. Each passing week away from Tina eased my stress; I looked forward to her finalizing the divorce.

On the fifth of June my mailbox held a thick envelope from the Seattle VA. I was elated. I was scared.

I walked into the apartment and poured myself a mug of coffee and sat down and had a cigarette. I trembled. I sweated. The time had come again and I was still not used to it.

I withdrew the pages from the envelope and the cover letter fell to the floor, leaving me holding the written copy of the official transcript of the hearing. That was nice; this time I had a written copy instead of a tape too garbled to understand. I figured the letter on the floor said something like, "Here is your copy of the transcript. The final decision for your claim will be sent soon."

I was mistaken.

> Dear Mr. Lewis:
>
> Following your personal appearance before the hearing officer at the Seattle Department of Veterans Affairs (VA) office on March 12, 1990, your case was carefully reviewed. That independent review by the hearing officer addressed not only your testimony at the hearing but a complete review of all the other evidence currently of record.
>
> The evidence of record including the testimony at the hearing and the additional evidence submitted since the last rating decision was given careful consideration by the hearing officer but no new basis was shown for assigning an evaluation in excess of 30 percent for your service-connected Crohn's Disease. Preparations will now be made to forward your records to the Board of Veterans Appeals in Washington, D.C. for their con-

> sideration. However, before this is done, consideration will be given to your claim for a total rating by reason of unemployability.
>
> If you have any specific questions concerning the outcome of your hearing, please write or call this office.
>
> A copy of the transcript of your hearing is enclosed, per your request.

So what the fuck is new? Nothing; just another thirty-second decision. Just another notification that I was in for another year of fussing and fighting with an incoherent and illiterate bunch of idiots. Even after doing their work for them, after quoting their own regs by chapter, page, and verse.

I put the letter down and took a long walk around the apartment complex. I beat some fir trees until my fists turned to bleeding raw meat. Every tree I beat on was Alan and Dave and the jerk who signed the letter. But fists are no good; I wished I had a chain saw.

I didn't expect to win on every point, but I expected to win at least one, for Christ sake! But as before, they didn't even *consider* all the issues; the letter referred only to the upgrade. It made no mention of retroactive awards. If "all" the testimony and evidence were considered as the letter claimed, then why was that issue left off the final decision?

Dave didn't even sign the decision, nor did anything on or with the document indicate he dictated it, read it or even approved it. Is this another case of one person conducting a hearing and someone else making the decision?

I showed Stan and Rob the transcript. Transcript — what a joke. It ran over with errors and inconsistencies. Responses were out of context or incomplete. Some questions weren't even on the record. How in the name of heaven could anyone use this information to make such an important decision?

I would seek a confrontation with the key players in this joke of a decision. I asked Stan if he would go with me and give me a hand at trying to talk some common sense into these morons. He said he certainly would.

I called the VA to, as the letter said, get answers to some "specific questions." I had questions, all right, a whole bunch of questions. Of course the letter had no phone number, so I called the switchboard.

"You are not allowed to talk to anyone in Adjudication," said Switchboard.

"I received a letter which said, and I quote, 'If you have any specific questions ... please write or call this office.' Now I am answering that invitation and I would like to be put through to the adjudication department as the letter instructs."

"I'm sorry, but we are not allowed to give out that phone number. Put your questions in writing and mail them."

"If I am not allowed to call, why is this statement included in the decision? Now please connect me with someone who can think." Then I mumbled as if to myself, but clearly enough for Switchboard to hear. "No damned wonder you people are as popular in the veteran community as the clap."

Switchboard repeated her order to write a letter, then the line went dead.

I called again, reached a different person, asked her to connect me with Adjudication. Same.

As I hung up the second time, my eye caught a little statement at the bottom of the letter:

America is #1 — Thanks to our Veterans

I called Alan. I told him I was not a happy man. I told him why.

He just said, "Umm-hmm. Well, tell me your specific questions and I'll try to get your answers."

"Nope. Not now. I am indeed going to put it in writing. To you. Please recall I stated at the outset I will hold you personally responsible for the outcome of this decision. You'll get my letter within a week."

For the better part of a day I labored over that letter, and it was pretty damned restrained given the rage that was consuming me.

> Dear Alan:
>
> This case with the VA has gotten totally out of control and beyond reason. It has exceeded nine and a half years with little justification. There is very little doubt in my mind that for whatever the reason, the VA has no intention of addressing my claim in a fair

and rational manner. They have consistently ignored the facts presented in this claim.

They have now placed themselves in a position of having to create reasons for denying my claim, based on being ignorant of issues already resolved in my favor. Their traditional response is, "If you don't like the decision file another appeal." That response is nothing short of a cop-out on their part, knowing that I must file another that will take another year and a half to get resolved, or hope I drop the issue entirely. Which will not happen!

I have gone well beyond the necessary requirements to substantiate my claim and they have absolutely no evidence counter to mine. I have even provided statements from a doctor who states I am 75 to 100 percent disabled. Yet the VA continues to deny me my entitlements with absolutely nothing contrary to the evidence I have provided. According to CFR Title 38, I have far exceeded the requirements of presenting my claim.

In 1981 I tried to explain that this problem would or could possibly affect my ability to work, but I was effectively ignored until it actually happened, and I lost my last job in 1986. Then I told them that it was affecting my marriage, and again I was ignored to the point that I was legally separated in February 1989, and my divorce is now pending. The last thing I have left is maybe I can salvage visitation rights with my daughter, but that will only happen if we can get this case resolved in my favor, so I can afford a lawyer to represent me. I have lost everything as the direct result of this damned disease and the VA continues to play ignorant. Of course none of this affects any VA personnel, so why should they care or give a damn. They have their jobs and a reasonable income.

I am trying very hard to maintain a modicum of dignity and reason with all this, but a person can only take so much. You can bet that if the VA chooses to continue to deny my claim I will take it all the way not only to the BVA but also to the new Court of Ap peals if necessary. As it now stands this regional office is wrong and is going to be embarrassed with the end result.

I feel that my claim is just and reasonable, and I am willing to compromise in order to get this finalized and over with. In an effort to provide the regional office an opportunity to save face and undue headaches, I respectfully request that you set up a meeting with the following individuals:

Director of Seattle VARO
Chief of the Adjudication Department
Alan Green (You)
Charles Lewis (Me)
Stan McCormik (Personal friend)

You coordinate the meeting with the VA people and let me know when and where to meet and I will be there and bring Mr. McCormik. The entire premise of this meeting is to resolve this claim once and for all, and walk out with a final decision that is fair and just.

Failing a fair effort on the part of this regional office and the necessity of returning to the BVA, I will file a formal complaint with the Secretary of the Department of Veterans Affairs and request his personal intervention through political means. I do not intend this as a threat of any kind. It is simply that I am tired and wish to get this claim resolved.

The delinquent manner in which I have been treated has already cost me much more than anyone would be willing to give up. Not to mention that it has essentially confused almost everyone involved. I will admit that the difficulties I have experienced are due equally to the disease itself and the lack of cooperation of the VA.

I am tired of going hungry the last third of every month. I am about to lose all contact with my daughter because of my ex-wife's vindictiveness and my inability to represent myself at my upcoming divorce hearing. I have already had the experience of being homeless and would rather not go through that again. I am really being pushed here, and I don't feel I deserve it.

Please set up the meeting I have requested if you are unsuccessful in obtaining a resolution to my claim within the next week. The last nine and a half years have been more than an ample, fair and reasonable amount of time for the VA to pull their collective heads out of their asses.

I really hope we can get settled without any more delay.

Sincerely,

CHUCK

There is serious need for major scale restructuring of the VA and in my ongoing journal I chronicled them all along. Now I noted another. Why doesn't the VA meet with the veteran as soon as the decision is made, and at this meeting, face to face, give him or her the decision, and spell out *reasons*. Allow the veteran the opportunity to challenge the decision immediately. Especially if the adjudicator overlooked or misconstrued any facts of the case. If warranted, many decisions could be "adjusted" (in case the VA wants to use that word instead of having to assume an implied error in being "overturned") on the spot without the need for further appeals. This would save the VA tens of thousands of dollars per claim, and it sure would save individual human beings years of agony.

Another point of reform so obvious a kindergartener could think of it would be to have the tape recordings of hearings transcribed in house, on premises, within hours. The presiding officer could review the transcript while the hearing is still within the range of human memory, and hand down his decision within the same millennium as the hearing.

By streamlining the procedure, issues actually get resolved, taxpayers' money doesn't get wasted, and the veteran doesn't spend the whole rest of his life jumping through the VA's hoops and loops. Or get tired of jumping and simply commit suicide.

Monday morning I poured the letter down the mail slot.

Tuesday afternoon Alan called. He said: (A) He liked the letter. (B) He sent it upstairs to the director of the regional office. (C) He, Alan, would "jump on the retroactive issue if I get the chance to talk to someone about it."

"Make the chance," I told him. "*You* go to *them* and *you* open the subject."

"All right. After that, the next move is up to the director He's sure to respond within a week.."

Thursday afternoon I answered the phone.

"Chuck? This is Alan Green, the American Legion Service Representative. Am I speaking to Charles A. Lewis?"

"Hi, Alan. This is Chuck."

"Sit down. Are you sitting down?"

Oh, shit, here we go again.

I told him I was seated. Then he dropped his bomb.

"Retroactive entitlement for the Crohn's disease at the rate of 30 percent has been approved back to the original filing date of 15 Jan 81, and you are to disregard the decision letter dated 1 June 90. Another letter reflecting this change will be sent shortly."

Then I was no longer seated. "Oh, Alan! Thank you, thankyou thankyou!" I gibbered. I saw some serious back pay coming, I saw all my bills paid, an attorney winning me custody of Andrea, a real car that really runs. Alan was trying to tell me something but I was having too good an orgasm to process what he was saying. Finally I settled down.

"We're scheduling you for a physical at Seattle VA Medical Center," Alan told me. "The hearing examiner needs an official update on your condition. Chuck, I'm going to tell you in capital-letters-underlined: Get to that physical! Your disability upgrade depends on it."

"In other words," I said, "my case is not closed. It is reopened."

"Right. A brand-new look at the whole ten yards. Evaluations for Crohn's *and* PTSD. And Chuck. Please, PLEEZE ... don't lose control with the doctors. Please don't swear. Please don't call them morons."

At my earliest meeting with Alan, he had suggested I arrange to get a physical, that the results might help my case. I declined, telling him if the hearing board wants a physical, the board can arrange for one. If I requested a physical on my own it would take four or five months before I actually got it. The hearing officer, on the other hand, could get the appointment in a matter of days. So that which I foretold had come to pass.

Aware that I had no wheels, Alan told me to let him know if I needed transportation to the physical. I told him I would get a ride somehow, somewhere.

Finally — a service rep who *did* something! Telling him I held him personally responsible — maybe I painted him into a corner. Which I meant to do. Or maybe he saw I had a good claim and went for the gusto. What I know for sure is: This guy took the VA to the wall and nailed them to it.

Where were you nine and a half years ago, Alan?

43

I called Ted in New York to share my good news, then Tim at The Hook. I called Stumpy, Jay, and Jack — separately. "Want you guys to get the word out the way it really happened," I told them. "Not grapevine-embellished."

When each of them advised me not to go out and buy anything yet, I answered them all the same: "If this has to go any further, Stumpy's going to go there with me."

Two weeks later I received the official decision. I found it pathetically comical the way the VA tried to cover its tracks. Damage control all over the place. The stiff, almost incomprehensible bureaubabble phraseology I found even funnier.

> Dear Mr. Lewis:
>
> Following our letter of June 1, 1990, your records were again reviewed by the Hearing Officer. It was noted that our earlier decision did not adequately address the evaluation of your gastrointestinal disability prior to your reopened claim in March of 1987. The second review took cognizance of the Board of Veterans Appeals' decision which originally granted retroactive service connection to an effective date of January 15, 1981. In that decision the Board conceded that the evidence of record was insufficient to establish the existence of Crohn's Disease, but was sufficient to establish service connection for idopathic colitis, based on the evidence available at the time of the original decision to deny benefits.
>
> After consideration of the evidence available to the original decision makers, consideration of your statements concerning this condition on review examinations for other disabilities conducted in 1983 and 1986, and the testimony presented at your Hearing in

> amplification and clarification of the course of your problems, it has been decided to award you benefits at the thirty percent rate effective January 15, 1981. Rating to implement this decision will be taken in the very near future and you will receive separate notice concerning the effect on your award benefits.
>
> This constitutes a substantial grant of the benefits you sought without appellate review. If our action satisfies the purpose of your appeal, you need do nothing further and your appeal will be withdrawn. If, however, you are not satisfied with this decision, you must tell us you wish to continue your appeal within 30 days of this letter. If we do not hear from you within 30 days of the date of this letter, we will consider your notice of disagreement and appeal withdrawn.

The letter of denial had arrived on the fifth of June. The letter award letter came on the nineteenth. On the twenty-second I got notice of my appointments for the medical exams: July 3 for Crohn's, the fifth for PTSD. I bet this is the fastest the VA has acted in the whole history of the world. Getting the physicals meant my case was still alive. It meant that for once I am not being avoided. It meant that for once a service rep was doing his job.

Rob and I went to Mike's for what we expected would be our last visit with that great and wonderful man. He was bedfast, barely able to move. The dark veil of death had won the war and the spirit of light was waging one last battle before retreat. Mike was mentally alert, but I have seen that veil too many times not to recognize it now.

Struggling to speak, Mike left me with a murmured set of instructions. "Keep up the fight with the VA. Don't let them beat you. Stand up for other vets who need help. Put your experiences in a book and tell this country what is happening to you veterans. Your story is too important not to tell."

I nodded in promise.

Mike went on. "Would you two please see to it that my classroom gets named for me?"

We promised to do what he asked. Actually, we had already discussed that very thing; we had already decided to do that.

I had to do something I hadn't been able to since Vietnam. I had to let this man know I loved him and I had to say good-bye while he could still comprehend what I was saying.

Just before we left I kissed Mike on the forehead and gave him a light hug. "Good-bye, Mike, dear and valued friend."

Rob and I fought back the torrents and we rode back in silence and when I got home I closed my doors and grieved for my dear and valued friend.

On the morning of July 3, 1990 Ruth arrived to drive me to Seattle for my physical. We were about to leave when the phone rang. It was my bank.

They "just wanted to inform me" that the VA had direct-deposited a check in my account for the sum of $18,000 and change.

After forcing myself not to faint (this was months sooner than I expected), my first thought was of Andrea. Now I could afford to buy her plane ticket for her summer visit — I'd have to hurry on that; summer flees. I'd be able to go and see and do with her: a ferry ride, the zoo, Mt. Rainier. Now I could get a car and be independent.

I was so excited it took ten minutes to get coherent enough to tell Ruth what happened.

The doctor had me in and out in fifteen minutes. He sent me for blood tests and x-rays ... The End.

I left the medical center wondering what the hell was happening. The exam was more a Q and A session than a physical. The doctor was obviously in a hurry.

As soon as I got home I took out my journal and made careful and detailed notes on this so-called exam, in case I needed the information later.

Two days later, chauffeured by my mom, I reported to the shrink. I told him right out that I wasn't sure if the stress problems were the result of Nam, or nine years of bullshit from the VA. We talked about Nam, the Crohn's and how it affects my lifestyle and emotions, the ever-present specter of having an accident in public.

The psychiatrist did not shortchange me; I spent an hour and a half with him and he talked me through my records, through every step of my history. As he did so I found out that almost of half my time in Vietnam was not accounted for in the VA's records. The VA recognized my presence there but there was no record of what I did or where I was assigned. So I discovered one more half-assed record in the VA system. Is there no end to all this crap?

The two exams were confusing in their contradiction. The psychiatrist gave me a completely sympathetic hearing, with all due time and detail. The physician rushed me through, doing little more than verifying that I had a pulse.

May as well start preparing for another Appeals hearing, Lewis. I have been preparing. Everything is written in my journal.

Near the end of July 1990 Mike lost his fight with cancer. We who were close to him met in the classroom he dominated at Green River College.

When I first set foot in Mike's classroom, the walls were completely covered, years of projects by his students' projects. Front wall, current events. Left wall, the fifties and sixties. Right wall, modern Asia and the Pacific Northwest. Back wall, the Vietnam War. A person could major in history just by studying the projects hanging on those walls.

About a year before Mike's death, some instructors who shared the room began complaining. The stuff distracts students. Distracts teachers. It's aging and unsightly. Mike was trying to claim as his own what was supposed to be public province. Blah blah, yada yada.

We who were Mike's friends saw it as conflicts of turf and personality, and of an administration which saw Mike as a little too dedicated: bad example to set for other faculty, you know. Mike had no intention of removing his students' work. The administration was equally determined to see it all come down.

The conflict continued for two quarters. In the end they took the projects down, repainted the walls.

The day Mike died his friends met in his room and got all the old projects out of the back room and put them on the walls. Our tribute to Mike, our public testimony of what he meant to us.

We also laid plans to have this classroom officially dedicated in Mike's honor. Other colleges do this, but Green River only named things after administrators or trustees or donors of the right amount of money. No faculty member had ever been deemed worthy of memorializing.

The crowd showing up for Mike's memorial service over-flowed his room, spilled from the building, and was moved to the amphitheater outdoors. I was deeply touched and honored that Mike's lovely widow and his sons asked me to speak. They knew of our fantastic friendship and of the bond we shared. I told all who were present, including the media, that Mike's loss represented an awful loss to higher education, and to the furtherance of honesty in the truths of history.

Mourners made a point of checking out Mike's notorious classroom before they left. The re-covered walls in that room were our challenge to the administration that we wanted Mike's memory kept alive.

The administration never picked up the glove. In apparent lack of regard for the faculty, nothing has ever been done. By mid-decade there still would be no faculty member ever honored by that school.

44

August 16, 1990. Another fat envelope from the VA.

I hoped for the best — I always did — and prepared for the letdown — it always was. After so many years of that, the cynic dwelt in me, and it was awake now.

After an hour of mentally preparing myself for the ultimate letdown I felt ready to open the letter.

Service connection has been established for the following conditions:

CONDITION	PERCENT
Crohn's Disease	60 %
Post Traumatic Stress Disorder with Psychological effects of Crohn's disease	30
Residuals of foot injury	20
Lumbosacral strain with sciatic radiation and limitation of motion	20
Bilateral high frequency hearing loss	0

This award has been made to you with a combined evaluation of 80%. This combined rating is not arrived by adding the percentages of your disabilities but is computed in accordance with a combined rating table.

> The evaluation of your service connected disability(ies) is less than 100% disabling. However, you are being awarded payment at the 100% rate because you are unable to secure employment because of your service connected condition(s). If you resume employment, you must notify VA as soon as possible as it may affect your entitlement to continued payment at the 100% rate.
>
> You are awarded benefits as follows:
> (Schedule of monthly stipends from April 1, 1990 through 1999.)

God, oh God! It's over. I WON ! ! !

After I sobered up some hours later, I realized I had been running around my apartment and out into the parking lot hooting and yelling like a banshee or something. The neighbors must have thought I had finally and truly wigged out at last. I didn't care. They could think what they wanted. After nine and a half years of fighting for this I had the right to flip.

Stumpy was the first one I called, as he had been since I met him. He was glad he wouldn't be repping me after all at the new Court of Veterans Appeals, glad it was over, glad he didn't get the job.

I told him about the award allotments. My monthly sums were just a little over the government's "official guidelines" for poverty level, but for me they would be sufficient. I never asked for a free ride; I never expected to become accustomed to luxury.

I commented that the monthly amounts decreased over time. Stumpy explained that I received extra for a dependent child. We did the arithmetic, which confirmed that my monthly decrease of just over $200 was scheduled for the payday after her eighteenth birthday. So some of my money was hers. Beginning with the first check I got for this award, I sent Andrea two hundred and ten dollars every month. I have never missed a payment.

"But, Stumpy, by my research the effective date of the award, April first, is in error. By regulation the award is to commence on the date the individual files the claim, regardless of when the hearing takes place."

"You're right," Stumpy said. "CFR Title 38 is very explicit on that point."

"Right. I looked it up, noted chapter and verse. I should be getting an additional eleven hundred a month for seven or eight months worth of back pay," I said. "That is some serious money I don't intend to let slide. If it was only a couple hundred bucks I would let it pass, but not something closer to ten grand."

That one oversight, I figured, was the VA's version of one last test question. I planned to ace this test all the way. I called Alan, thanked him profusely, then gave him his last assignment: Correct the VA's arithmetic on the matter.

Two days later Alan called me with the news: The VA accepted that the date was in error, and corrected it.

Peace at last.

The relief of finally bringing to an end this fight with the VA was exhausting in its own right. After nine and a half years of filing, filling out forms, writing letters, being lied to, ignored, and stripped of all sense of personal dignity, it's finally over. I won, but in the process, I lost. I lost everything I own, including my family. I paid a very high price for this so-called victory.

Yeah, it's over, Lewis, but tomorrow starts the rest of your life. Look at it this way: You lost two people— a shrew and an angel. But you gained a whole fold of good and faithful friends, each of them a bar of gold-pressed latinum.

Right, Voice On My Shoulder. And for tomorrow and all the tomorrows after, I'll be fighting for all the other American veterans. So stay right where you are, and hold on for a hell of a ride.

AFTERWORD

I seriously question any system which feels it necessary to put an individual through what I went through for nine and a half years. This is the story of only one individual, yet these experiences are not uniquely mine. Other veterans have been treated worse, some not as badly. But whether their treatment is horrifying or merely abominable, is the conduct of the Department of Veterans Affairs acceptable to the people of this country?

To say that the government is your best friend while you serve it, and your biggest enemy when you are no longer its servant is . . . a pretty fair assessment as I see it.

The commitment I made to myself was this: I would not quit; I would not give up. I refused to allow the VA to strangle me in red tape or to chase me off with its hostility, indifference, and incompetence. But I am one of relatively few. Tens, perhaps hundreds of thousands of veterans have simply given up, or worse, they committed suicide because of the inaction of the agency that was created to care for them. Though I did not withdraw my request for the benefits legally due me, I did lose everything that was important to me: a family I loved; my livelihood; my self-esteem, dignity, and pride.

I did not write this as a Boo-Hoo story or for self enrichment, but rather, to try to bring home some truths and help correct some terrible wrongs. Americans see the angry veterans on the streets of their nation but they don't understand the anger. I hope to enlighten those who do not know. I hope to inspire other vets to get back into the battle — to fight for what is legally, ethically, and morally theirs. To claim what our nation promised them.

If this nation does not keep its promises, what will the future hold for those who serve it? We will have no military! Who would be willing to serve?

On the surface, the war in Vietnam, in and of itself, did nothing to jeopardize our system. Or did it? Those dedicated enough not to run from the call did some very dirty work in the name of this country, and they paid a very heavy price. Promises were made which turned out to be worth less than the paper they were written on. The agency charged with the responsibility of caring for those dedicateds is quite possibly the earth's biggest morass of hindrance and non-cooperation. While all the socialist programs of post-Vietnam rampantly mushroomed (often in favor of those who ducked out), veterans saw their share of the pie decrease until there was practically no pie at all.

VA health care facilities have curtailed their services and diminished their quality of health care delivery. Many have been partially or entirely closed down, increasing the burden on those that do remain open and are already overwhelmed. Waiting six months or more to get a basic medical appointment is not unheard of.

After dedicating twenty or more years to their nation's defense, retirees are not getting the free health care they were promised.

Military retirees are the only group not allowed to concurrently collect full retirement *and* full disability pay.

VA guaranteed home loans have been downgraded. A veteran can get a better deal by going down to the corner Mortgage Company, saving himself thousands of dollars.

Many of those promises are broken in the name of deficit reduction, balanced budget, and national debt. But I submit to you that this nation incurs more debt in maintaining an incompetent system than it would in dispensing justice. It costs far less to pay a man his due than to care for him via welfare. To award him what he has been promised is cheaper than keeping him in prison.

Things have changed very little in recent years. In the spring of 1993, the Acting Deputy Director of Benefit Programs for the VA went before the United States Congress to request permission to conduct the arbitrary and wholesale denial of over 600,000 pending disability claims. The request was the agency's effort to clear VA employee's desks of all backlogged files. Does this demonstrate our government's contempt for the veteran community? Does it show how important veterans are to an administration headed by a draft-dodging president? Then too, there is the question of why there are so many backlogged cases to begin with. Would it have anything to do with party planning and donut-dunking breaks, or to sheer mismanagement and incompetence?

Congress turned down the request, but the fact that there existed the audacity to even approach lawmakers with such a reprehensible proposal speaks of the government's contempt for its veterans. Of course, the VA always includes the polite notation that those whose claims are denied can always re-file. How thoughtful. No big deal, though: re-file-appeal-wait only adds a mere year or two to the years a vet's case has already been on hold. What about doing it right in the first place? How's that for a novel idea?

We cannot accept excuses about national debts and budgets. Our country made a contract with those who serve. Nowhere did it refer to its being a fair weather obligation. It is a contract that must be honored. Period, end of sentence. Yet as recently as July 1997, a Congressman asked for $27 million to give to India. Reason: to protect the Indian Elephant, which is now on the endangered species list. How many vet centers could be kept open with that kind of money? How many homeless veterans' shelters could that kind of money support?

I recently heard a guy complaining that because of budget cuts, his free drug rehab center was closing. Since when is it the taxpayers' responsibility to pay for his addiction? If he can afford to buy drugs, he can afford to pay to learn *not* to buy them. Doing drugs was his choice, not the taxpayers'.

The stories of stupid, frivolous, wasteful use of tax dollars go on and on. NO, lack of money is not a valid or honest excuse for the betrayal of America's veterans.

Mr. President and members of The Congress, if you cannot honor your obligations, if you refuse to pay your bills, do not send this nation's youth out to do *your* dirty work! The ordinary citizen who breaks a contract is called a criminal. What makes you think you are not? It's commonly accepted that the words *honesty* and *integrity* do not fit in the same sentence as *politician*. I wonder why.

Two positive steps have been taken. The Court of Veterans Appeals (COVA) is in place. Veterans are now allowed to pay attorneys a fee that's decent enough to attract lawyers to represent them. But there still is much to do.

Forming a cabinet-level Department of Veterans Affairs was a good try and an honest effort, but it is not the answer, either.

The rampant problems, the scheming and indifference are at the local level and therefore not within the normal observation range of highest-echelon offices in Washington, D.C. Corruption is apparently not reportable to higher authority; it is covered up at the Regional level because regional officials fear exposure will make them look inept. Besides, ineptitude has continued for so long that the public thinks of it as standard procedure.

I am not about to leave the National Veterans Service Organizations (NVSOs) out of this, either. They need to do some serious housecleaning, themselves. It is abundantly clear that all the veterans' organizations must work together instead of working in their own little domains, protecting their own provinces. Veterans' groups are so divided that the Congress and the DVA capitalize on that divisiveness to further their own personal self-interests.

What, pray tell, makes any one organization better than others? Technology changes the battlefield, but fire, lead, and steel still violate the human body and leave permanent marks, regardless of the name of the marks. "Shell Shock" or "Post Traumatic Stress Disorder" still deprive one of a normal life.

In the final analysis, what does it matter which war, conflict, peacekeeping mission, or police action an American is called to? It is time to stop arguing about which was a "real" war and to recognize instead the bonds that unite all warriors. It is time for veterans' service organizations to *serve* veterans, instead of politicking, colluding with the DVA, bending to lobbyists, and giving up veterans' rights for the sake of bigger game.

There is no feasible way the government could have gotten away with what it has done all these years if all the NVSOs really did what they claim to do, namely, represent this country's 26.5 million veterans and protect their interests. It would be almost impossible for us to lose benefits in the way we are now if your groups would simply work together.

Veterans Service Organizations, you complain you are losing membership numbers, and you wonder why. Let me enlighten you! You betrayed the grassroots veterans. They no longer see *you* as representing *them*. They see you as merely one more cog in the "D.C. Beltway Mentality." The veteran community *would* rally around you, provided you would assume some leadership and get back to the job at hand.

The first and foremost solution to the veterans' problems is this. The hostility and indifference of the Department of Veterans

Affairs must stop, and it must stop now. Our leaders in Washington must try really hard to remember that they are in office because 26.5 million men and women sacrificed to make sure our leaders *have* a country to lead. Failure to treat the veterans they serve with dignity, respect, and honest effort should be grounds for the immediate dismissal of any public servant, whether elected, appointed, or an entry-level hireling.

The nation desperately needs to establish an entity to oversee the ethics and conduct of the Department of Veterans Affairs. A roving inspection team must have the authority to drop in on any Regional Office to monitor and audit every aspect of its operation. The team must have the authority to fire any individual who does not meet standards of conduct and productivity. It is time to stop the career building on the back of those guardians of our democracy who need the democracy's help.

Drug testing of all DAV employees, including supervisors, should be mandatory and frequent. Verified users of illicit drugs should be fired automatically and immediately. Further, supervisors should be fired if they are aware of underlings' abuse of drugs but fail to take action. Consider what I observed in New Jersey.

The DVA must be required to send claim-related documents by certified or registered mail. Not knowing if a veteran received correspondence from the VA is absolutely inexcusable. As a Federal agency, the VA is entitled to free use of the government franking stamp; therefore sending documents by certified mail incurs no extra costs to the agency.

The Court of Veterans Appeals must be reorganized so that it carries the authority of a real court. As it exists, the VA system can keep individuals in the appeals process for years before the case ever works up to the COVA. Then if the COVA finds any error or miscarriage, the court can only return the case to DVA "for further review." That the COVA is one step past last resort speaks for the sluggishness, lack of justice, and extravagant wastefulness of the whole system.

Claims must be processed faster. The whole file hearing-appeal-start over process could be streamlined by several steps and dozens of bureaucrats if it permitted the veteran to be present during the first stages. As the system is, everything that is supposedly done on the veteran's behalf actually transpires in secret, as if the veteran is an enemy agent.

As the system is, in fact, it seems more an employment agency than a servant of the people. All the stalling, subterfuge, losing things, covering up; all the shuffling of claimants from one person, one office, one "part of the process" to another; all the not knowing anything, the butt-covering and damage control; all the starting over — these keep a lot of workers occupied. To vets like me who have been through the system, it seems as if for every $1000 appropriated to the DVA, $990 goes for nice buildings and bureaucrats' salaries, and $10 is awarded to the veterans whose claims keep them employed. American taxpayers would have been saved tens of thousands of dollars if my own claim, to cite only one example, had been handled properly in the first place.

Since few of those solutions are likely to be put in place very soon, here's a simple, pragmatic, practical one: Put a warning label on recruitment offices and enlistment papers. Warn all who would join that they may very well not get what the military promises them.

I firmly support a strong, healthy military force. Our nation's position in the world depends on it; without it our status would be significantly diminished. However, when a nation — any nation — has a military, that nation is obligated to honor its commitments to those who serve in it.

I cannot advocate anyone's joining the military today. Overall, I enjoyed my time in the service and I served with pride. But those in our armed forces cannot count on entitlements and benefits their government promises but may rescind at a moment's notice. Once they are sworn in, members of the military accept their obligation under penalty of law. But if by its double standard the government no longer wants to honor its obligations, it simply ignores them — or changes the law. If America sees fit to continue its revocation of contracts made with those who serve, eventually our youth will get wise and not volunteer to enlist.

Realistically, what can be done? Possibly nothing. Yet if there was enough of an outcry to our national political leaders, maybe the needed reforms would be made. Veterans would like to see the rescinded promises reinstated. All we ask is simple justice. No more, no less.

If we fail to honor our commitments to those who serve, we will no longer have anyone willing to serve. Then what would we do?

about the author . . .

Long an active leader in veterans' affairs in the state of Washington, Chuck Lawrence has gained notability nationwide as a spokesman for Vietnam veterans throughout America.

One of the founders of VVA Chapter 690 (Auburn, Wash.), Lawrwnce served as its vice president, president, and public speaking chair. For three years he was Legislative Coordinator for Washington State Council of VVA. He was a four-year member of the Washington State Veterans Legislative Coalition, serving a term as its Co-Chair.

He received a gubernatorial appointment to the Governor's Vocational Rehabilitation Advisory Committee, where he represented Washington veterans.

His involvement in bringing the Vietnam Memorial Traveling Wall to the Pacific Northwest was one of Lawrence's most rewarding projects. He counseled, supported, and was just there for fellow veterans encountering the Wall for the first time.

Nationally, Lawrence was appointed National Interim Commander for VETS, a new organization which seeks unity within the veteran communities and addresses Congress regarding the loss of veterans' benefits and entitlements.

Lawrence lives near Seattle.

A seasoned public speaker and presenter, Chuck Lawrence speaks and teaches at schools, college classes, civic and service organizations, and public events.

To inquire about a presentation, e-mail Y34@aol.com.

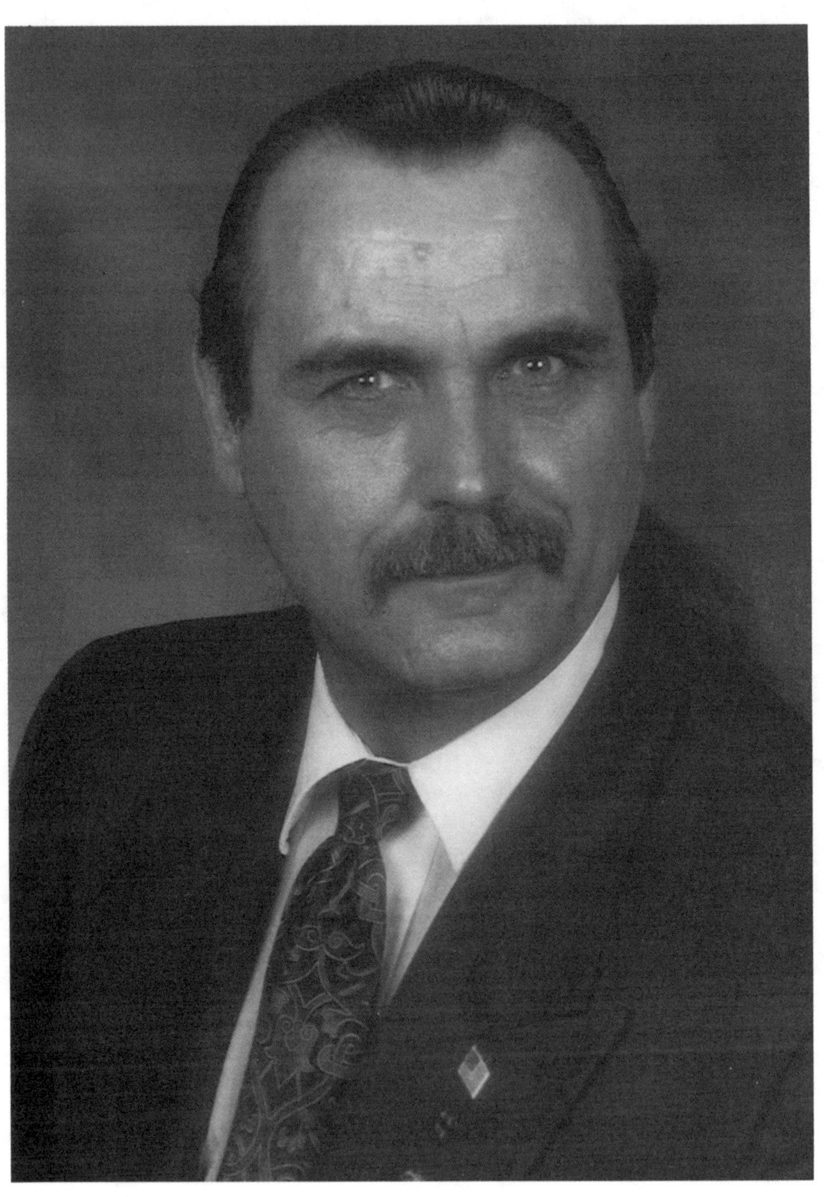

ORDER FORM

Name ____

Address____

City/State/Zip_______________________________________

Phone____

TEARS OF BLOOD (paperback)_______________$19.95

TEARS OF BLOOD (hardcover)_______________$24.95

Shipping/Handling____________________________$3.50

Washington State residents add 8.6% sales tax

Send to Soaring Eagle Publishing
P.O. Box 2536
Auburn, WA 98071-2536